Little Recipe Book

Culinary Secrets *from a* Lebanese Kitchen

IKBAL JOSEPH

© 2022 Ikbal Joseph and Suzanne Joseph
All rights reserved. No part of this book may be reproduced or used in any manner without the prior written permission of the copyright owner, except the use of brief quotations in a book review. Send permission requests to littlerecipebook@use.startmail.com.

Compiled and translated by Suzanne Joseph
Copyedited by Carrie Wicks and Thomas Berger
Exterior Book Design by Damonza
Interior Book Design by Van-garde Imagery
Recipe photographs by Ikbal Joseph and her family members
Author photographs by Haissam Masri
Translator photograph by Michele Sutherland

Nutritional information was calculated with an online recipe calculator. Nutrition details are only rough estimates. They are not intended as dietary recommendations or medical advice.

ISBN 979-8-9851412-2-1 (Hardcover)
ISBN 979-8-9851412-5-2 (Paperback)
ISBN 979-8-9851412-9-0 (eBook)

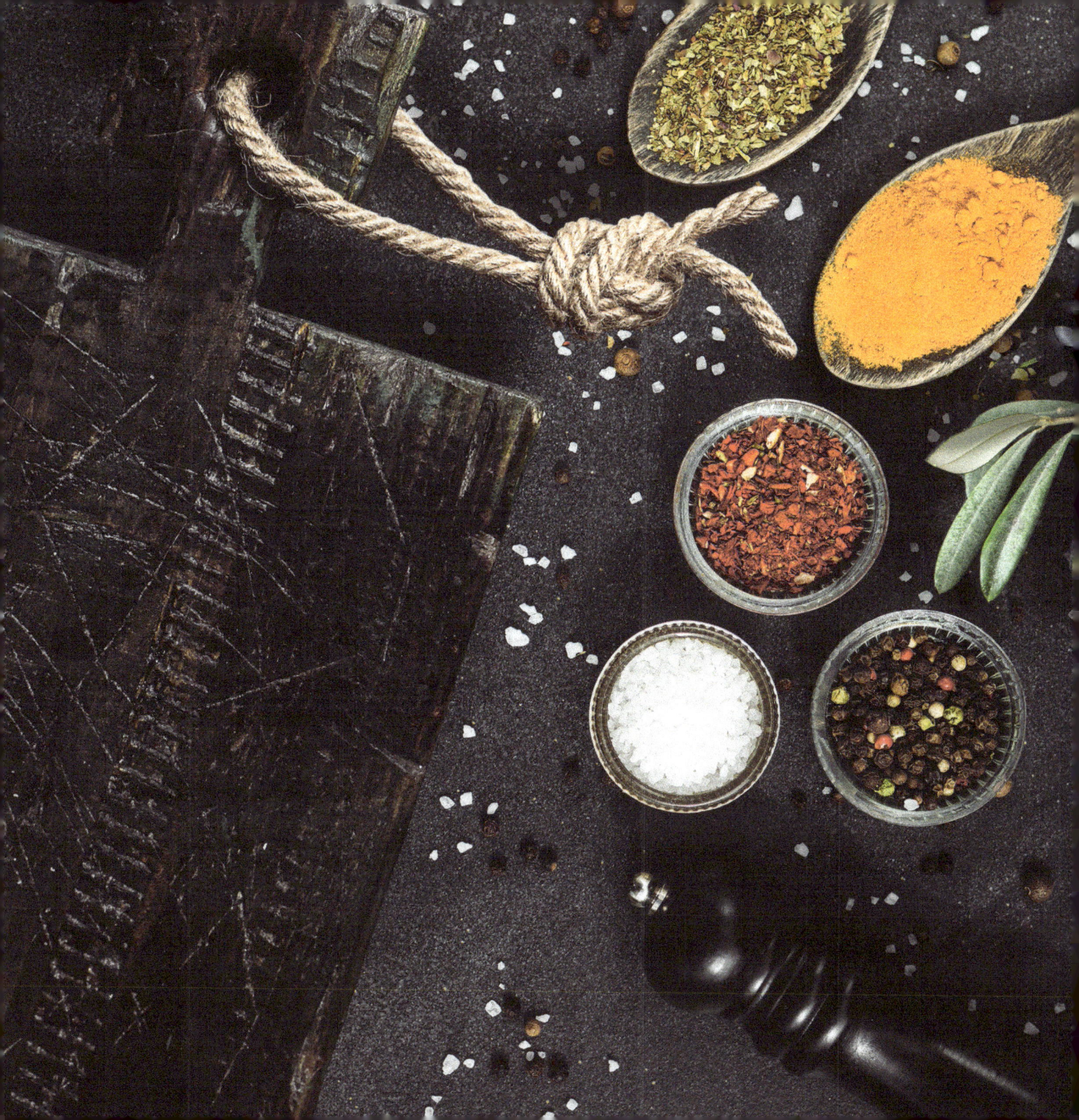

Contents

Foreword   vii

Introduction   ix

Meze & Salads

Hummus   2

Roasted Eggplant Dip *(Baba Ghanoush)*   4

Lentils with Rice *(Mujadara)*   6

Falafel   8

Lebanese Salad *(Fattoush)*   10

Parsley Salad *(Tabbouleh)*   12

Stews

Jute Mallow with Chicken *(Molokhia bi Dajaj)*   16

Okra and Meat Stew with Rice *(Bamia bi Lahm ma Riz)*   20

Lima Beans and Meat Stew *(Fasolia bi Lahm)*   22

Pea Stew and Rice *(Yakhni bi Bazella ma Riz)*   24

Green Bean Stew *(Loubieh bi Zayt)*   26

Lentil Stew with Swiss Chard and Lemon *(Adas bi Hamoud)*   28

Stuffed Vegetables & Vines

Stuffed Grape Leaves with Meat *(Warak Enab bi Lahm)*   32

Stuffed Grape Leaves without Meat *(Warak Enab bi Zayt)*   36

Stuffed Cabbage Rolls *(Warak Malfouf Mahshi)*   40

Stuffed Cousa Squash *(Cousa Mahshi)*   44

Stuffed Cousa Squash with Yoghurt Sauce *(Cousa Mahshi bi Laban)*   46

Artichoke Bottoms Stuffed with Meat *(Ardishowki bi Lahm)*   50

Eggplant Stuffed with Meat *(Sheikh el Mahshi)*   52

Meat, Poultry & Fish

Baked Kibbeh   56

Kibbeh with Yoghurt Sauce *(Kibbeh bi Laban)*   58

Garlic and Pepper Kafta   61

Classic Kafta   62

All-Spices Kafta   64

Sweet and Spicy Kafta   66

Lebanese Lamb with Rice   68

Lebanese Spaghetti with Béchamel *(Macaroni bi Halib)*   70

Beef Shawarma   72

Chicken Shawarma   74

Lebanese Chicken and Rice *(Riz bi Dajaj)*   76

Lebanese Chicken Wings   78

Spicy Fish *(Samaki Harra)*   80

Lebanese Fish with Rice *(Sayadiya)*   82

Fusion Dishes

Stuffed Mushrooms   88

Lebanese Lasagna   90

Eggplant Parmesan   92

Lebanese Shepherd's Pie   94

Ikbal's Citrus Chicken   96

Desserts

Lebanese Rice Pudding *(Meghli)*   100

Lebanese Sweet Cheese Pastry *(Knafeh bi Jibn)*   102

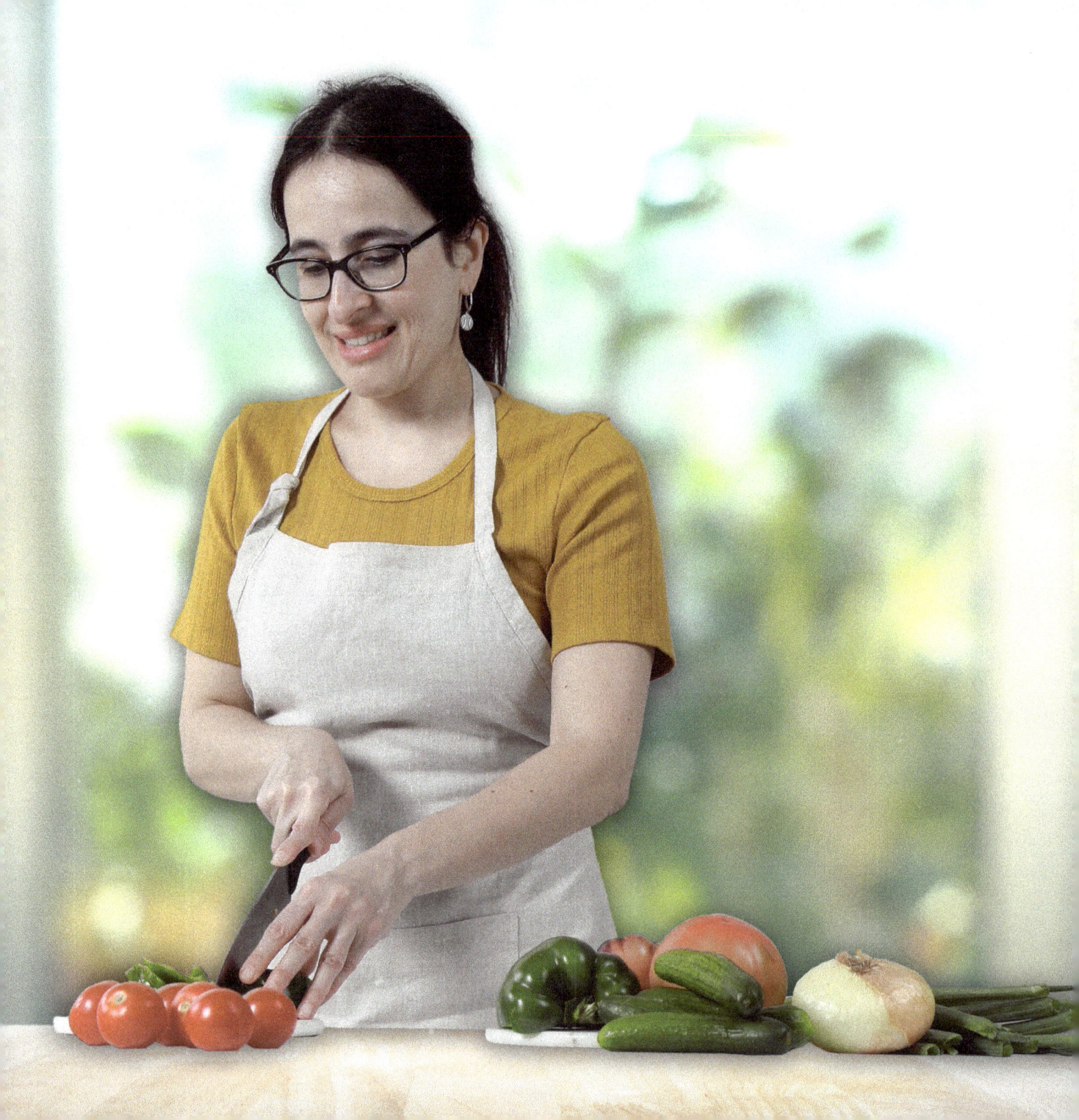

Foreword

The mission behind the *Little Recipe Book: Culinary Secrets from a Lebanese Kitchen* is simple: to help you prepare food of unparalleled taste that you, your family, and friends will enjoy year after year. The recipes may seem exotic, but they are easy to follow and bring a healthy indulgence to any kitchen.

How did the *Little Recipe Book* come about? The author, Ikbal Joseph, was born in Lebanon and began cooking when she was nineteen years old. Because she loved good food and grew up in a cooking culture, she watched, tasted, and started putting together her own recipes of traditional Middle Eastern dishes. Ikbal loved cooking for others and, by doing so, developed a growing following wherever she went. From early on, intensity of flavor and versatile seasoning became hallmarks of her cooking.

Since immigrating to the United States from Lebanon in 1970, she has divided her time between the two countries, eventually opening her own restaurant in Sarasota, Florida, on world-famous St. Armands Circle.

Although Ikbal has retired from working as a professional cook, she has never stopped cooking at home. She currently spends her time honing tried-and-true recipes, developing new ones, and tending her fruit and vegetable garden.

For years, Ikbal has heard the same frustrations voiced over and over by fans seeking her advice: "My dish just didn't taste as good as yours. What are your secrets?" In response, she decided to put together this recipe book containing her most popular recipes with secret cooking tips that make each recipe special. As one of her most ardent followers (who happens to be her daughter), I was delighted to help compile these recipes, translating some of the finer points from the original Arabic.

Ikbal believes that fabulous food bursting with flavor should be within everyone's reach. The *Little Recipe Book* brings the tastiest Lebanese cuisine directly to your kitchen. Read. Cook. And enjoy!

—Suzanne Joseph

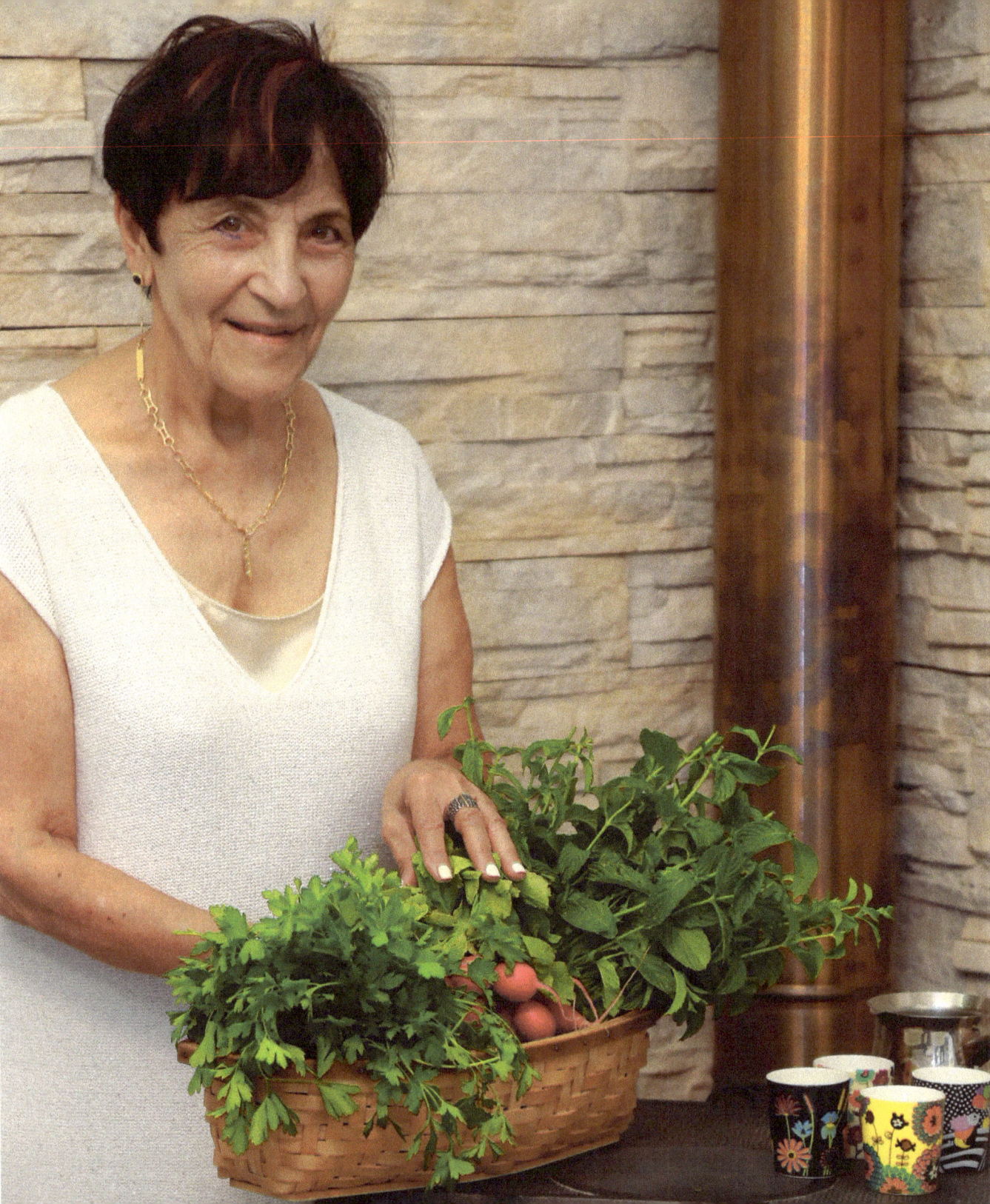

Introduction

Cooking is a unique convergence of work and pleasure. There is no denying that cooking requires a great deal of concentration and focus. That is why it's important to put yourself in a positive frame of mind before you begin cooking. Set the mood by pouring yourself a cup of coffee or other beverage of your choosing. Put on some music and clear your mind. And, remember, a clean and organized kitchen will make your task easier.

Rest assured that Lebanese food is well worth the effort. The recipes contained here are rich in flavor and full of fresh herbs and vegetables as well as assorted spices that will keep your palate happy. Each of these dishes, too, is a visual feast that can be enjoyed not only for its pleasing taste and aroma but for its aesthetic presentation. Combining ingredients in a recipe is like mixing colors on a palette or knitting together different strands of yarn.

The cooking and sharing of food is also a form of communication just as important as language. Defining moments in our lives are made especially memorable with wholesome, great-tasting food. I remember serving Lebanese rice pudding (*meghli*) to friends and family after the birth of each of my three children. It's a longstanding tradition among different religions in Lebanon to prepare the pudding in celebration of a newborn baby. Some groups also serve the pudding on birthdays and religious holidays. Our family tradition was to serve it to all guests who came to visit and offer their congratulations within the first forty days of the child's birth. Nothing brings people together and strengthens relationships like great food, especially pudding!

Most of the recipes that follow are classic Lebanese dishes that I've prepared for years. Some are a fusion of Lebanese and other culinary traditions. All the recipes were selected by popular demand, either by former restaurant patrons or a small cooking circle of family and friends. Each recipe comes with one or more photos, a list of ingredients with corresponding step-by-step instructions, key tips, and nutrition information.

I hope that you enjoy preparing these recipes for many years to come.

With best wishes,
Ikbal Joseph

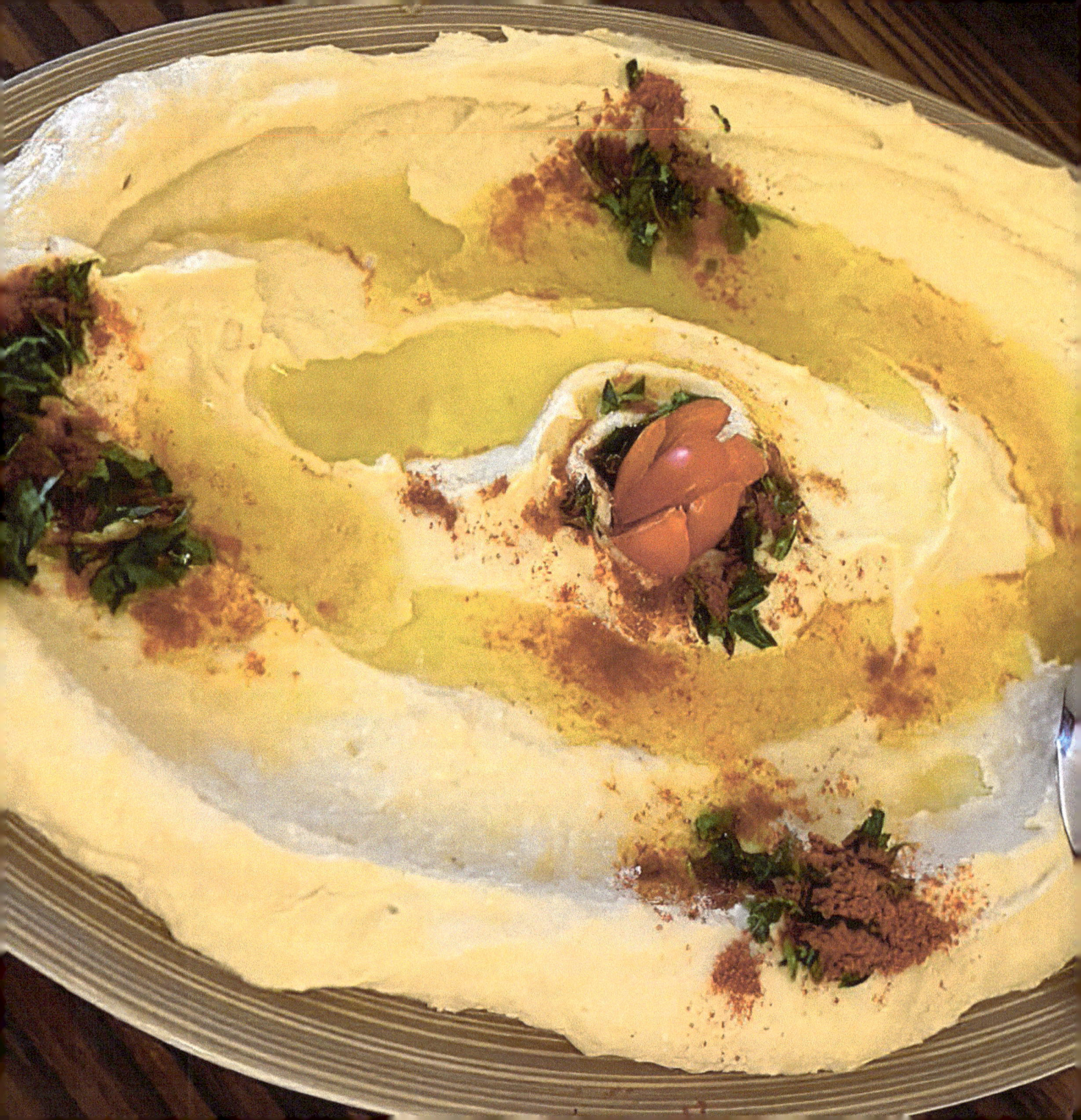

Meze & Salads

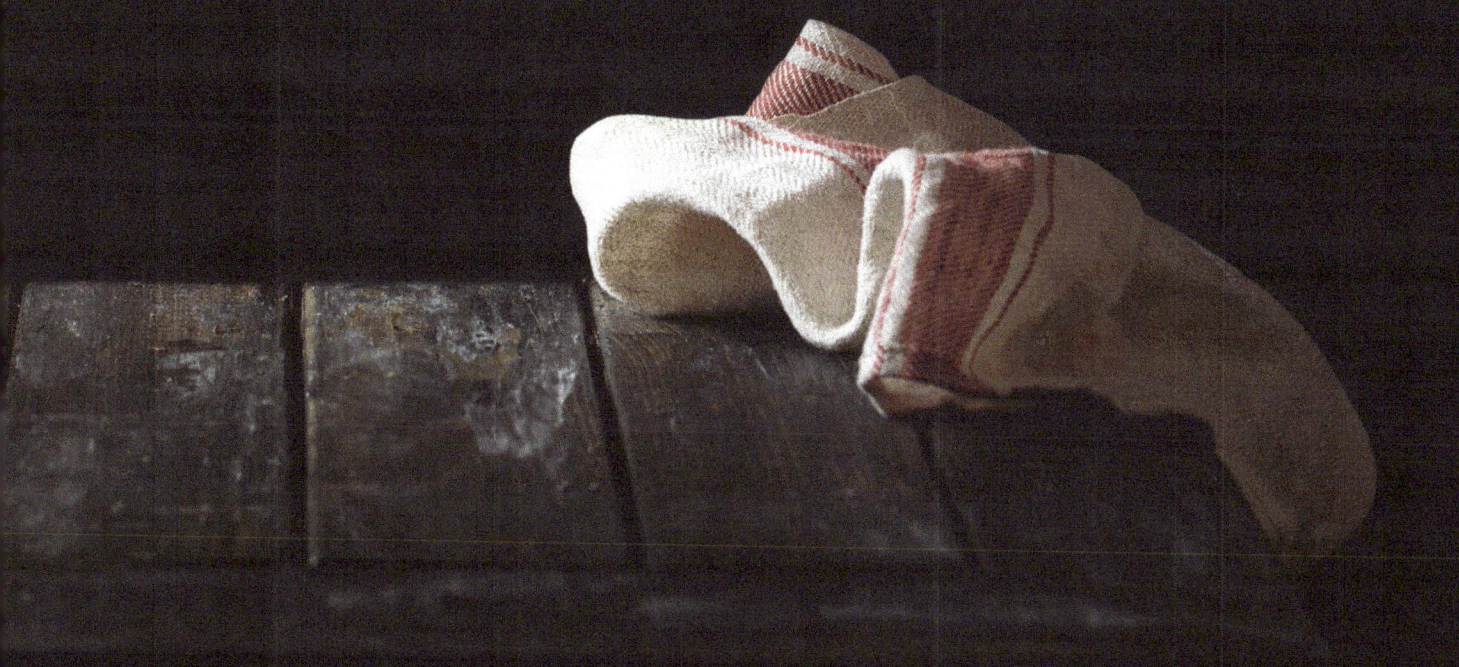

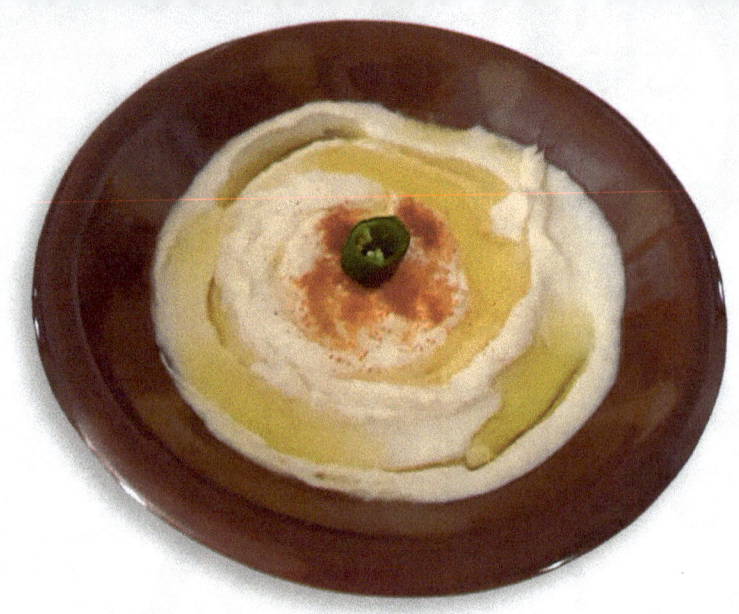

HUMMUS

Serves 4–6
Total time (preparation & cooking):
30 minutes + 12 hours soaking

---

nutritional information per serving (4.8 oz.) **Cal** 482 **Fat** 18.8g (sat 2.4g) **Chol** 0mg **Carbs** 62g **Sugars** 10g **Protein** 21g **Fiber** 12g **Sodium** 274mg **Vit. A** (4% DV) **Vit. C** (17% DV) **Calcium** (11% DV) **Iron** (29% DV)

INGREDIENTS

1	pound dried chickpeas or garbanzo beans (may substitute with canned chickpeas)
6	cups water
2	tablespoons baking soda
½	cup lemon juice (freshly squeezed or bottled)
½	teaspoon table salt
3	garlic cloves, peeled and crushed
4	tablespoons tahini (sesame paste)
2½	tablespoons extra-virgin olive oil
½	teaspoon paprika (optional)

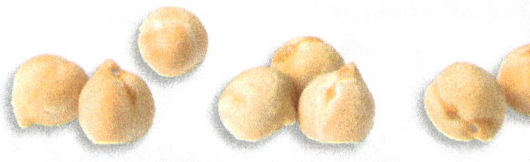

INSTRUCTIONS

1. **Soaking the chickpeas:** Place the dried chickpeas or garbanzo beans in a large bowl. Fill the bowl with enough water to cover the chickpeas. Add the baking soda and allow to soak for 12 hours. When complete, strain the chickpeas and discard the soak water. Rinse the chickpeas with tap water, using a colander to strain.

2. **Cooking the chickpeas:** In a large stockpot or rondeau with about an eight-quart capacity, bring the water to a boil and add the chickpeas. Cook on a low boil for 1 hour and 30 minutes, or until the chickpeas are tender. Cover after about 15 minutes to allow time to spoon off any white foam that forms on the top of the water. Halfway through cooking time (at about the 45-minute mark), remove the cover and check that there is sufficient water to prevent the chickpeas from sticking to the pot or burning. Add water if needed.

   Strain the chickpeas using a colander, saving ¼ cup of the boiled chickpea broth. (If using canned chickpeas, do not soak or boil. Place chickpeas directly in a food processor or blender along with ¼ cup of liquid from the can.) Set aside a handful of whole chickpeas for garnish.

3. **Pulsing the chickpeas:** Using a food processor, pulse the cooked chickpeas with the saved chickpea broth for several minutes until a paste is formed. Add the lemon juice, table salt, garlic cloves, and tahini. Pulse until well blended. Add 2 tablespoons of the olive oil and pulse again until smooth.

   Pour onto a serving plate. Garnish with whole chickpeas and sprinkle with paprika if desired. Drizzle the remaining ½ tablespoon of olive oil evenly over the hummus.

   May be served as is or with pita bread.

   Cook's secret: Blend the chickpeas with broth first, and add the extra-virgin olive oil at the very end.

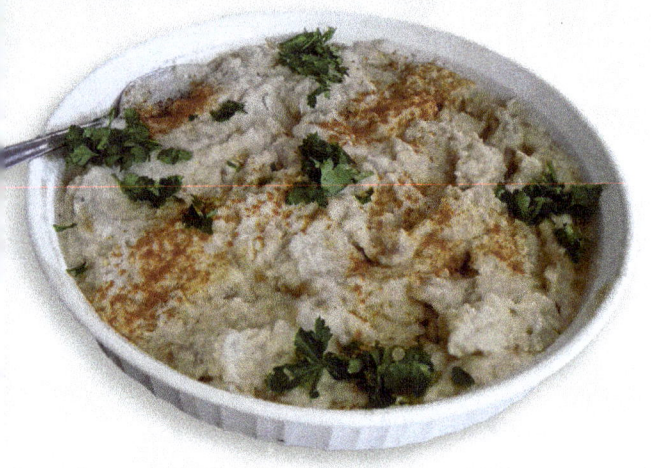

ROASTED EGGPLANT DIP
(BABA GHANOUSH)

Serves 4
Total time (preparation & cooking): 1 hour

---

nutritional information per serving (5.6 oz.) — **Cal** 94 **Fat** 5.3g (sat 0.8g) **Chol** 0mg **Carbs** 11g **Sugars** 5g **Protein** 3g **Fiber** 5g **Sodium** 159mg **Vit. A** (1% DV) **Vit. C** (13% DV) **Calcium** (5% DV) **Iron** (7% DV)

INGREDIENTS

- 1 large eggplant
- 2½ tablespoons tahini (sesame paste)
- 1 small garlic clove, peeled and crushed
- ¼ teaspoon sea salt
- 1 large lemon, freshly squeezed
- ½ teaspoon paprika (optional)

INSTRUCTIONS

1. **Preparing the eggplant:** Roast the eggplant on the stovetop or grill on high heat, turning it over regularly to ensure even cooking. Once the eggplant is tender and a knife can easily slide into the fleshy center, cut it in half, lengthwise. Using a spoon, remove the cooked center and place it in a large glass or ceramic bowl. Mash the eggplant with a pestle or spoon to break down and soften. Add the tahini, garlic clove, and sea salt. Mix well to combine. Add the lemon at the end and mix again. Top with paprika for garnish if desired.

May be served as is or with pita bread.

Cook's secret: Add the squeezed lemon at the very end.

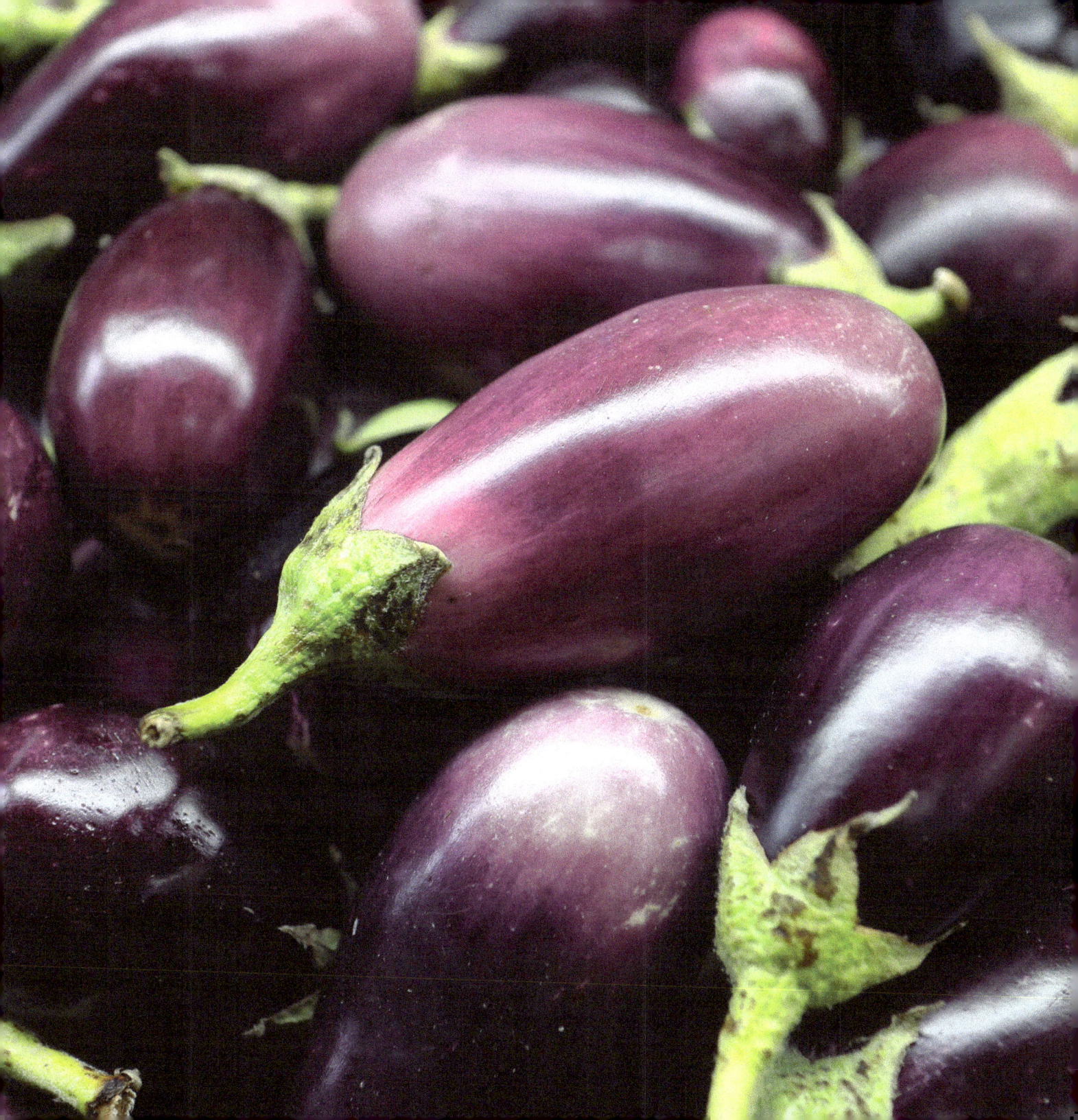

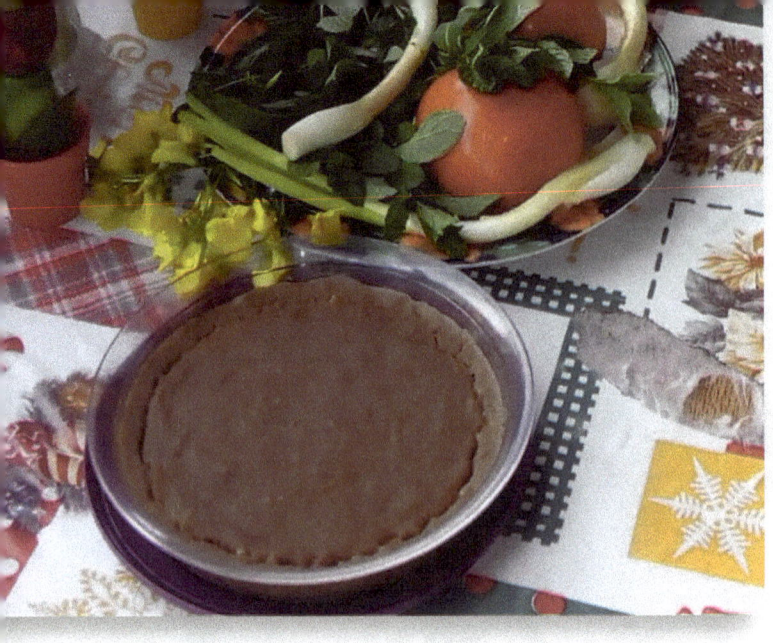

LENTILS WITH RICE
(MUJADARA)

Serves 4-6
Total time (preparation & cooking):
1 hour, 35 minutes

---

nutritional information per serving (13 oz.) — **Cal** 435 **Fat** 32.8g (sat 4.6g) **Chol** 0mg **Carbs** 29g **Sugars** 4g **Protein** 8g **Fiber** 7g **Sodium** 650mg **Vit. A** (0% DV) **Vit. C** (13% DV) **Calcium** (6% DV) **Iron** (18% DV)

INGREDIENTS

- ¾ cup extra-virgin olive oil
- 2 large white onions, diced (Vidalia onions preferred)
- ¼ cup medium-grain Egyptian white rice (may substitute with Arborio rice)
- 2 cups dried brown lentils
- 4 cups water
- ¼ teaspoon cumin, ground
- ¼ teaspoon black pepper, coarsely ground
- ¼ teaspoon allspice, ground
- 1 teaspoon table salt

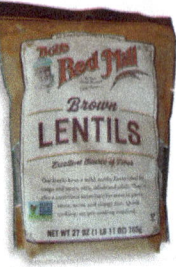

INSTRUCTIONS

1. **Preparing the onions:** In a frying pan, heat the olive oil and add the onions. Cook on medium heat for about 10 minutes, or until the onions turn golden brown. Set aside.

2. **Preparing the rice and lentils:** Rinse the rice, drain, and set aside. Sift through the lentils by hand to remove any hardened or shriveled pieces. Using a colander, rinse and drain the lentils. In a medium saucepot, bring the water to a boil and stir in the lentils. Reduce heat to low and add the cumin, black pepper, allspice, and table salt. Cover and cook the lentils on a low boil for 55 minutes, or until soft, adding the rice at the 30-minute mark. Stir occasionally to prevent lentils from sticking. When cooking time is complete, check the water. There should be about ¼ cup of water left in the saucepot. Add water if needed.

Stir in the prepared onions and cook with the lentils for another 15 to 20 minutes, or until almost all the water is evaporated. Onions and lentils must be stirred constantly while cooking. Pour contents onto a large plate and allow to cool. Serve at room temperature or store in the fridge and serve chilled without reheating.

May be served as is, with pita bread, or with cabbage salad (composed of half the head of a thinly diced cabbage, a couple of chopped mint leaves, 1 chopped tomato, 1 chopped small radish, juice from ½ lemon, 2 tablespoons of olive oil, and ½ teaspoon of table salt).

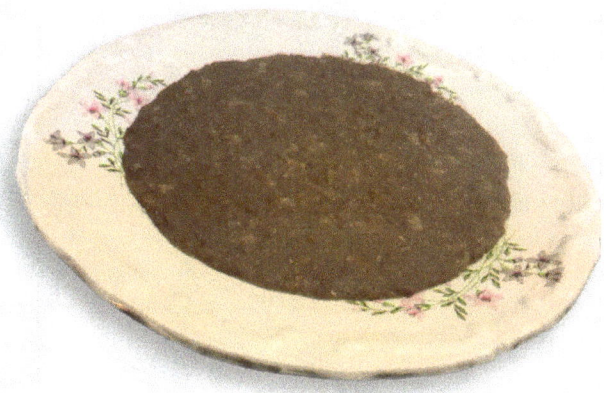

Cook's secret: Use large sweet onions and brown to caramelize.

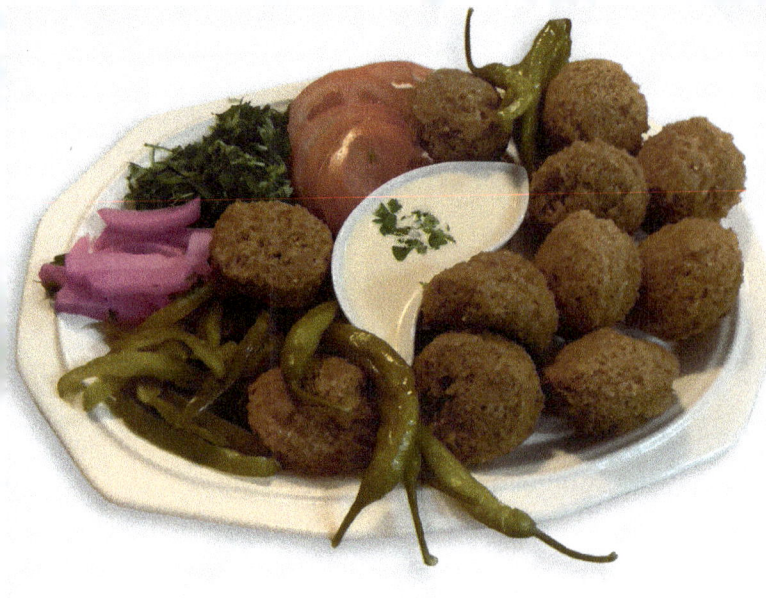

FALAFEL

Serves 4–6
Total time (preparation & cooking):
2 hours + 12 hours soaking

---

nutritional information per serving (5.8 oz.) — **Cal** 680 **Fat** 26.1g (sat 2.7g) **Chol** 0mg **Carbs** 83g **Sugars** 10g **Protein** 33g **Fiber** 29g **Sodium** 868mg **Vit. A** (4% DV) **Vit. C** (6% DV) **Calcium** (19% DV) **Iron** (47% DV)

Ingredients

- 1 pound dried, peeled fava beans
- ½ pound dried, peeled chickpeas or garbanzo beans
- 1½ teaspoons baking soda
- 1½ teaspoons baking powder
- 1 teaspoon sea salt
- ¼ teaspoon cinnamon powder

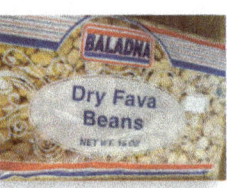
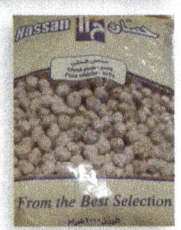

- ½ teaspoon dried cilantro
- ½ teaspoon garlic powder
- ½ teaspoon paprika
- ½ teaspoon black pepper, coarsely ground
- ½ teaspoon white pepper
- ½ teaspoon ginger powder
- ½ teaspoon cumin, ground
- 2 cups vegetable oil (sunflower oil preferred)
- 1 egg, lightly beaten (optional)

INSTRUCTIONS

1. **Soaking the beans:** Place the fava beans and chickpeas in separate water-filled bowls to cover the beans. Add 1 teaspoon of the baking soda to the bowl of fava beans and add the remaining ½ teaspoon of baking soda to the bowl of chickpeas. Stir to combine and allow the beans to soak overnight for about 12 hours. When complete, strain the beans and discard the soak water. Rinse the fava beans and chickpeas thoroughly with water using a colander. Drain well.

2. **Pulsing the beans:** Place the fava beans and chickpeas together in a food processor or blender. Pulse until the mixture is smooth with a gum-like consistency. Do not overmix.

    Remove pulsed beans from the food processor and place in a mixing bowl. Add the baking powder and sea salt. Mix slowly by hand. Add the cinnamon powder, dried cilantro, garlic powder, paprika, black pepper, white pepper, ginger powder, and cumin, using hands to gently combine the ingredients. Let the falafel sit in the fridge for 1 hour before frying.

3. **Frying the falafel:** Shape the falafel into small, rounded patties (somewhat larger than a golf ball, or about 2 inches in diameter). Heat the vegetable oil in a deep fry pan without a lid. Make sure that the oil is hot before adding the falafel patties. Drop one of the patties in the oil to test. If the falafel crumbles and does not hold its shape when frying, add the egg to the falafel mix, and stir to combine. Fry the falafel patties for about 2 minutes on each side, or until they turn golden brown. Remove from the pan and place in a colander, draining for several minutes. Place the falafel on a plate lined with a paper towel to absorb excess oil.

May be served as is or with fresh tomatoes, fresh mint, pickled turnips, and a tahini-based sauce, or *taratour*, in a pita sandwich.

Cook's secret: Use the specified 2:1 ratio of fava beans to chickpeas.

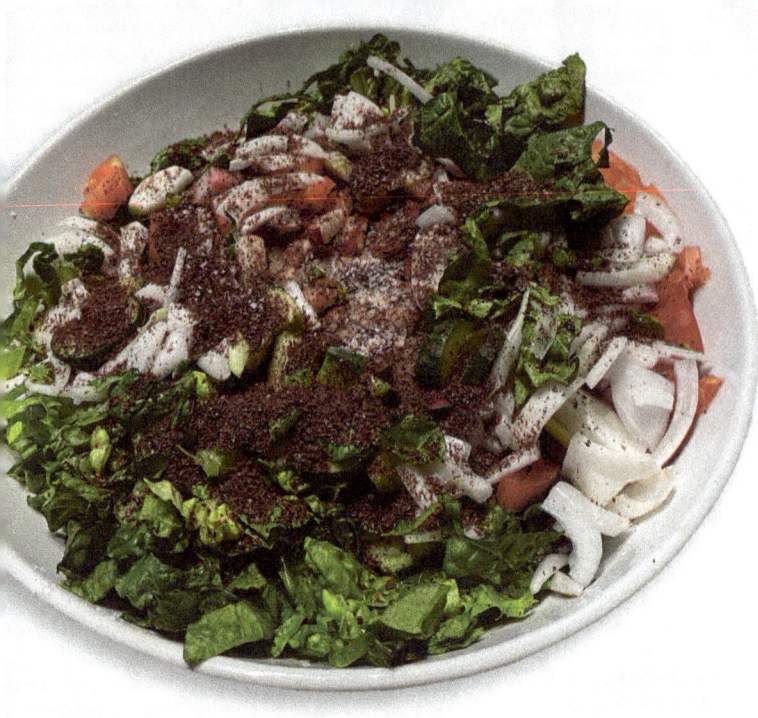

LEBANESE SALAD

(FATTOUSH)

Serves 4–6
Total time (preparation): 55 minutes

---

nutritional information per serving (13.1 oz.) — **Cal** 263 **Fat** 22.3g (sat 3.1g) **Chol** 0mg **Carbs** 15g **Sugars** 7g **Protein** 3g **Fiber** 4g **Sodium** 516mg **Vit. A** (83% DV) **Vit. C** (50% DV) **Calcium** (7% DV) **Iron** (11% DV)

INGREDIENTS

- 1 large garlic clove, peeled and mashed
- 1 teaspoon table salt
- 5 medium cucumbers, chopped in small pieces
- 2 medium tomatoes, chopped
- 6 large romaine lettuce leaves, medium chopped
- ½ sweet onion, cut into thin wedges
- 5 small radishes, chopped
- 1 bunch fresh purslane leaves, un-chopped (optional)
- 1 bunch fresh mint leaves, coarsely chopped
- ½ bunch Italian parsley, chopped with stems removed
- 1 large loaf white pita bread, toasted
- 1 medium lemon, freshly squeezed
- 2 heaping tablespoons sumac
- ½ cup extra-virgin olive oil

INSTRUCTIONS

1. **Preparing the vegetables:** In a large salad serving bowl, place the garlic in the base with the table salt. Add the cucumbers, tomatoes, romaine lettuce, onion, radishes, and purslane leaves.

2. **Soaking and draining the herbs:** Place the parsley (without stems) and mint in a separate bowl. Fill the bowl with water and let sit for several minutes. Drain using a fine mesh sieve. Repeat this process three times to remove all the dirt. Do not wash the parsley and mint prior to chopping as the herbs will end up wet and soggy. Once the parsley and mint are washed and thoroughly drained to remove excess water, add them to the serving bowl.

3. **Topping and dressing the salad:** Place the toasted pita chips on top of the herbs and vegetables. Add the lemon and sumac. When ready to serve, add the olive oil and toss the salad.

Best served as is.

Cook's secret: Use fresh mint in the salad and a generous amount of sumac.

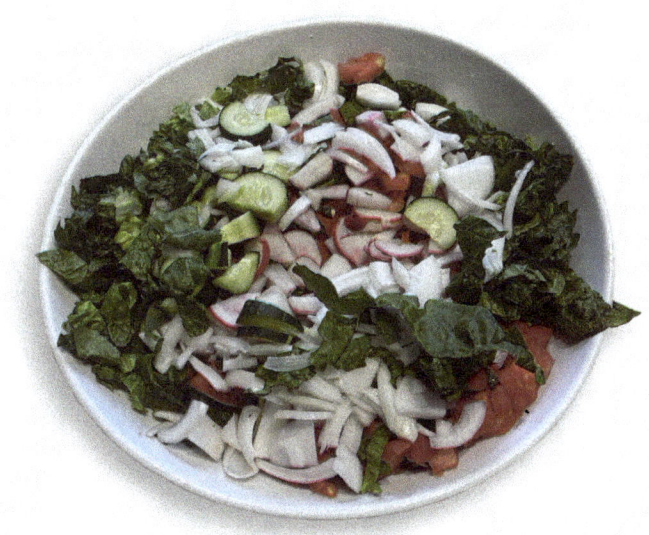

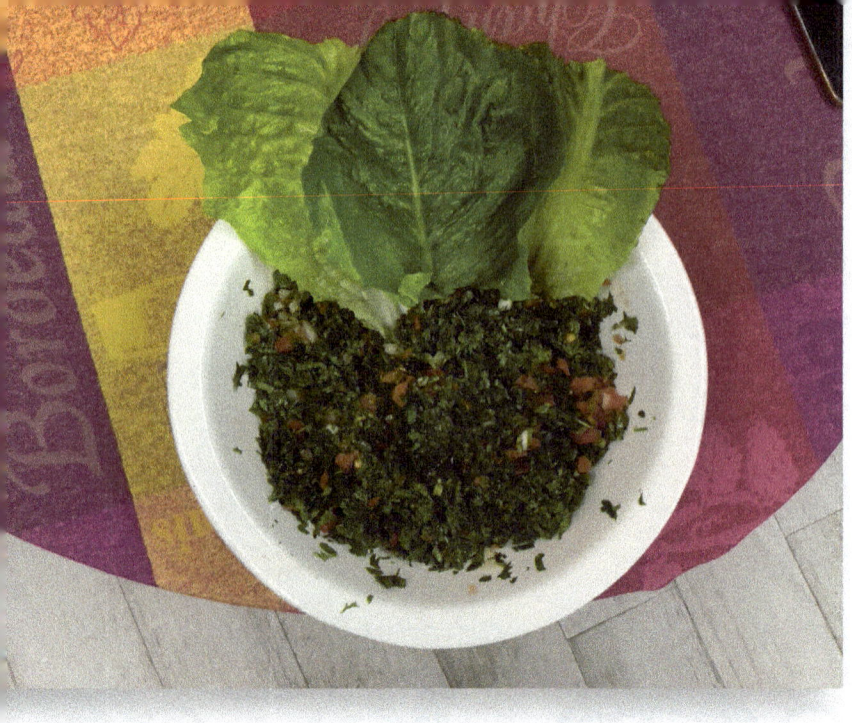

PARSLEY SALAD
(TABBOULEH)

Serves 4–5
Total time (preparation): 1 hour

---

nutritional information per serving (8.9 oz.) — **Cal** 304 **Fat** 27.7g (sat 3.8g) **Chol** 0mg **Carbs** 14g **Sugars** 5g **Protein** 3g **Fiber** 4g **Sodium** 323mg **Vit. A** (90% DV) **Vit. C** (132% DV) **Calcium** (9% DV) **Iron** (18% DV)

INGREDIENTS

- 1½ tablespoons fine bulgur (optional)
- 2 bunches (5.3 ounces) Italian flat parsley, finely chopped with stems removed
- ½ cup fresh mint, finely chopped
- 2 scallions, finely chopped
- 3 large tomatoes, finely chopped
- 1 small white onion, finely chopped
- 1½ lemons, freshly squeezed
- ½ teaspoon table salt
- ½ cup extra-virgin olive oil

INSTRUCTIONS

1. **Preparing the bulgur:** If using bulgur, soak the bulgur in water for 3 to 4 minutes to soften. Drain the bulgur in a fine mesh sieve and set aside.

2. **Soaking and draining the herbs and vegetables:** Place the chopped parsley (without stems), mint, and scallions in a large salad bowl. Fill the serving bowl with water and let sit for several minutes. Drain with a fine mesh sieve. Repeat this process three times to remove all the dirt. Do not wash the parsley, mint, and scallions prior to chopping as herbs and vegetables will end up wet and soggy. After the washed parsley, mint, and scallions are thoroughly drained to remove excess water, place in a medium serving bowl.

3. **Putting it all together and dressing the salad:** Add the tomatoes, white onion, bulgur (if desired), lemon, table salt, and olive oil to the serving bowl. Use hands (cleaned with unscented soap) to combine ingredients and ensure that the parsley is well saturated (with tomatoes, lemons, and olive oil).

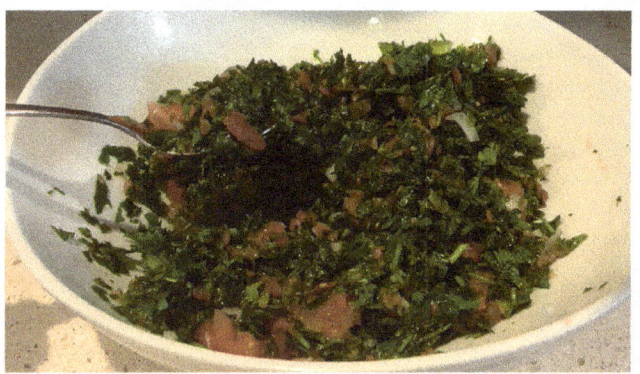

May be served with fresh cabbage, romaine lettuce, or grape leaves.

Cook's secret: Drain the parsley, mint, and scallions well, and mix the salad thoroughly by hand.

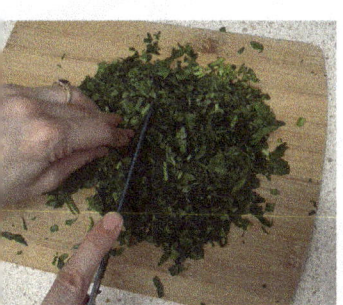 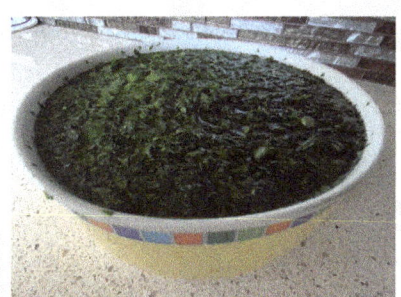 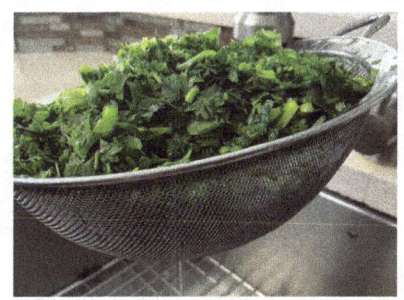 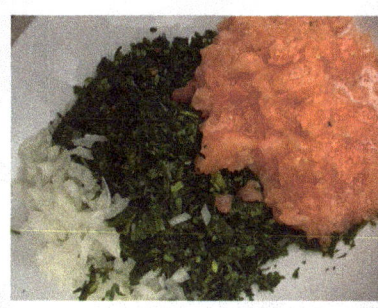

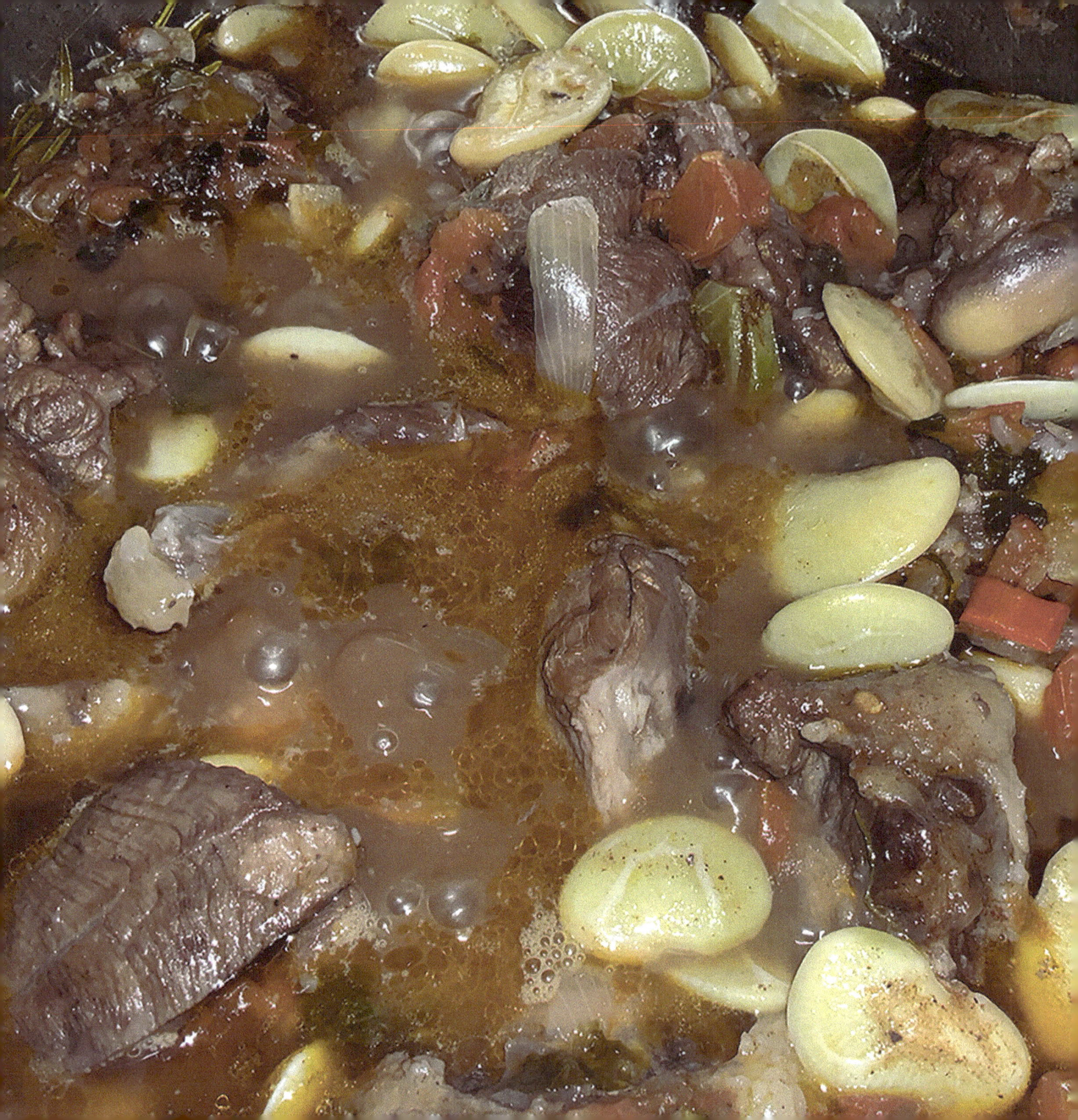

Stews

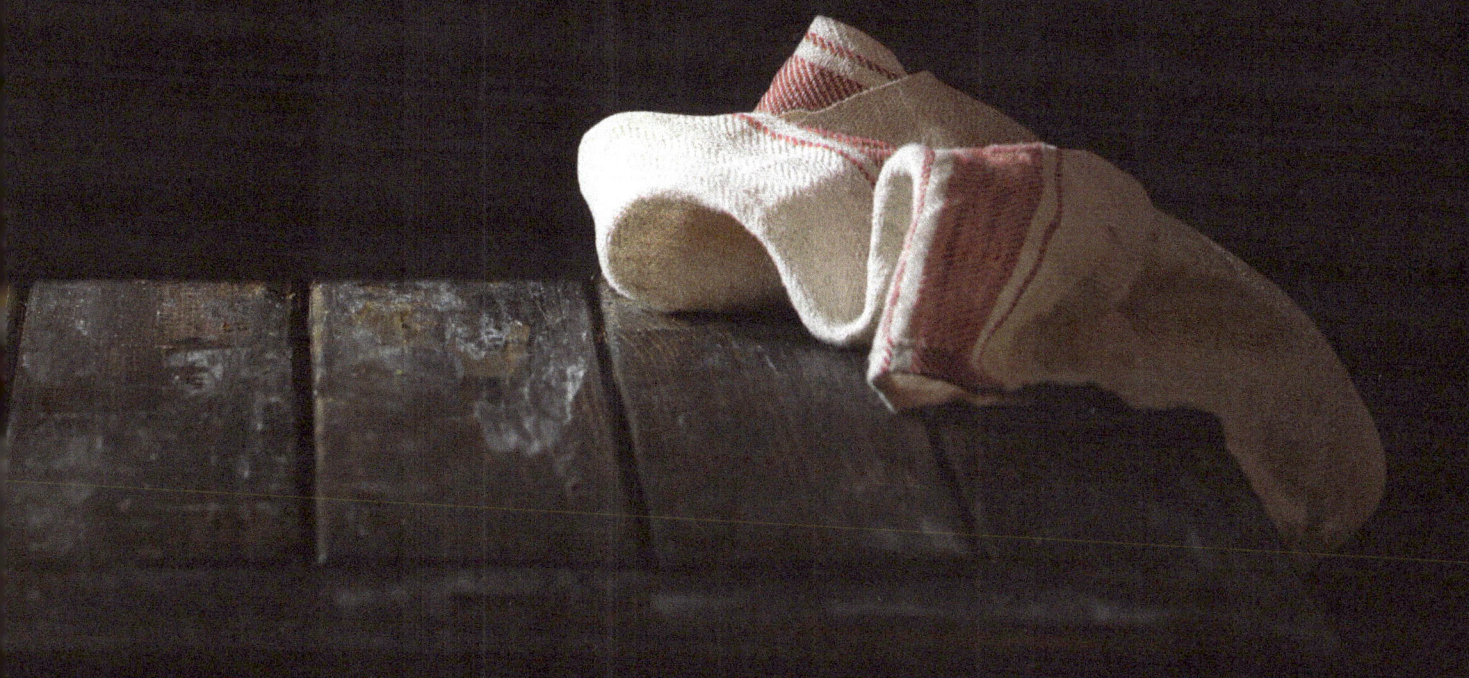

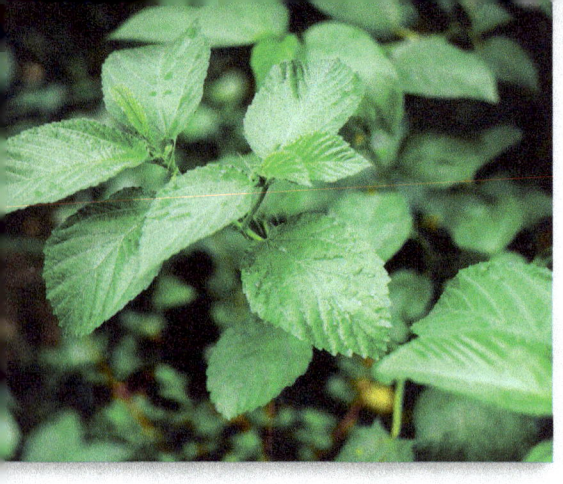

JUTE MALLOW WITH CHICKEN
(MOLOKHIA BI DAJAJ)

Serves 6–7

Total time (preparation & cooking): 3 hours, 40 minutes

nutritional information per serving (22.6 oz.)	**Cal** 674 **Fat** 41.4g (sat 11.1g) **Chol** 122mg **Carbs** 41g **Sugars** 12g **Protein** 40g **Fiber** 6g **Sodium** 1471mg **Vit. A** (165% DV) **Vit. C** (170% DV) **Calcium** (41% DV) **Iron** (54% DV)

INGREDIENTS

- 1 whole chicken (skin-on)
- 3 tablespoons all-purpose flour
- 1½ lemons, freshly squeezed
- 3 teaspoons table salt
- ½ teaspoon cinnamon powder
- 1 teaspoon black pepper, coarsely ground
- 1½ teaspoons allspice, ground
- 6 tablespoons extra-virgin olive oil
- 2 large onions, chopped
- 4 small onions, cut in half
- 19 garlic cloves, peeled
- 9 garlic cloves, unpeeled
- 1 tablespoon soy sauce
- 1 lime, halved with rind
- 4 bay leaves
- 4 cardamom, whole
- 4 cloves, whole
- 4 tablespoons red wine
- 7 medium onions, chopped
- 3 tablespoons unsalted butter
- 2 cups fresh cilantro, coarsely chopped
- 2 garlic cloves, peeled and diced
- 2 (14-ounce) packages frozen whole-leaf *molokhia*, or jute mallow, thawed
- ½ fresh hot pepper, diced with seeds removed
- 1 loaf pita bread (optional)

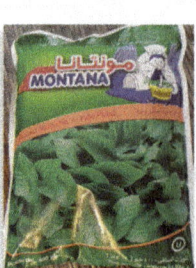

Vinegar & onion dressing

- ½ cup red wine vinegar
- 2 small onions, finely chopped
- ½ fresh hot pepper, diced with seeds removed (optional)

INSTRUCTIONS

1. **Preparing the chicken:** Scrub the chicken with the flour, ½ squeezed lemon, and 1 teaspoon of the table salt. Rinse thoroughly with cool water. Allow the chicken to dry. Spice the chicken by adding the cinnamon powder, black pepper, allspice, and the remaining 2 teaspoons of table salt.

2. **Cooking the chicken:** In a large stockpot or rondeau with a height of no less than 6 inches and a five-quart capacity, cook the chicken with 3 tablespoons of the olive oil on low heat. Turn the chicken on all sides, adding the chopped onions and the halved small onions. Stir and continue to cook until the chicken turns golden brown. Add 8 of the peeled garlic cloves (unchopped), the soy sauce, and the halved lime with rind. Cook for several more minutes. Pour water over the chicken so that it barely covers the chicken or reaches about 2 inches below the top of the stockpot. Bring to a boil and reduce heat to low-medium. Add the unpeeled garlic cloves, the bay leaves, cardamom, and whole cloves. Stir in 2 tablespoons of the red wine.

   Cook the chicken for 1 hour and 30 minutes on low-medium, or until it is cooked through.

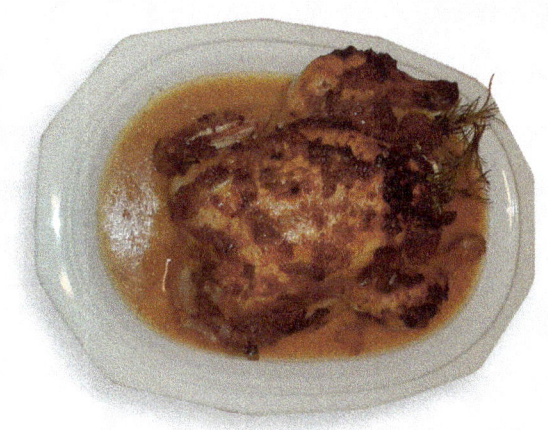

3. **Deboning the chicken and saving the stock:** When cool enough to handle, carefully remove the cooked chicken meat and skin scrapings, placing them in a covered food storage container. Shred the chicken by hand into medium-size pieces. Make sure to remove all the chicken from the bottom of the pan, along with any caramelized skin. Add some water to ease the removal of chicken scrapings if needed. Discard the bones. Cover the stockpot, saving the liquid chicken stock with cooked onions and unpeeled garlic for the molokhia stew.

4. **Preparing the roasted onions and garlic:** Place 7 of the peeled garlic cloves (unchopped) in a food processor or blender. Pulse once or twice to break them up into large chunks. Set aside. Place the (chopped) me-

dium onions in a baking pan. Roast in a preheated oven at 350°F for 15 minutes. Add the pulsed garlic chunks to the baking pan and roast together with the onions for 5 minutes. Remove the roasted onions and garlic from the oven and place them in a food processor. Pulse twice so that the garlic and onions remain chunky in consistency. Set aside.

5. **Preparing the cilantro:** Heat 1 tablespoon of the olive oil and 1 tablespoon of the butter in a small pan on low. Add 1 cup of the fresh cilantro. Stir for a minute or two. Then add the diced garlic cloves to the pan. Sauté together on low-medium heat for 5 minutes. Set aside.

6. **Cooking the *molokhia* stew:** Remove the thawed molokhia from packages and drain well to remove excess water. Cook the molokhia on medium heat in a separate stockpot or rondeau with a minimum four-quart capacity. Add the remaining 2 tablespoons of olive oil and 2 tablespoons of butter. Cook for about 20 minutes. Add the remaining squeezed lemon and 1 cup of fresh cilantro (uncooked). Gently lift and turn the ingredients to fold or combine, taking care not to overmix. Add the hot pepper and the remaining 4 peeled garlic cloves (unchopped) to the molokhia. Cook for several minutes before folding in the prepared cilantro and the prepared roasted onions and garlic. Add the remaining 2 tablespoons of red wine.

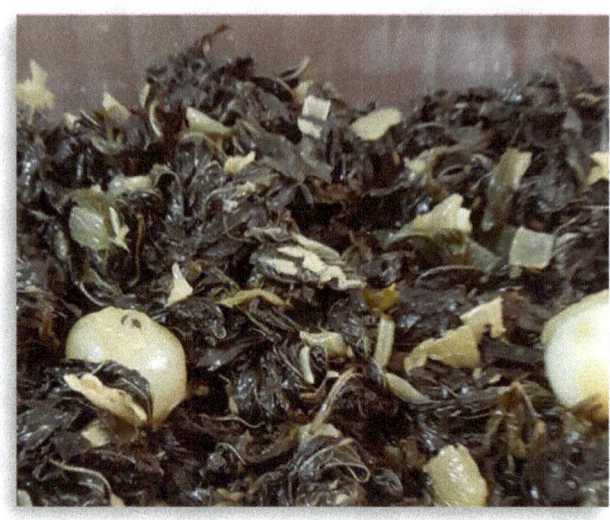

Remove about 2½ cups of the liquid stock from the chicken preparation and gradually add it to the molokhia. If there is insufficient chicken stock left, add water instead. Remove each of the 9 (unpeeled) cooked garlic cloves from the liquid stock and squeeze each clove out of its skin into the molokhia, discarding the skin or peel.

Do not add the cooked chicken to the molokhia stew since the chicken is best served separately. Cook the molokhia covered for 1 hour on medium-low heat, reducing heat to low for the last 20 minutes. Remove from the heat after molokhia has cooked for a total of 1 hour and 20 minutes. Keep covered. Serve hot or warm.

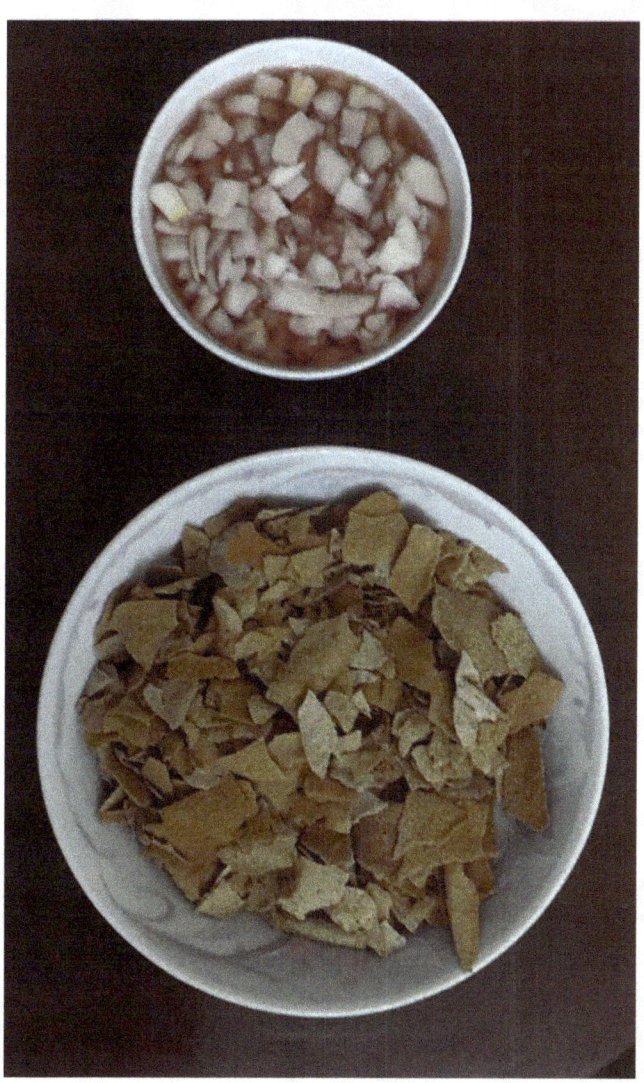

7. **Preparing the vinegar-and-onion dressing:** In a small bowl, combine the red wine vinegar, onions, and hot pepper (if desired). Set aside.

8. **Putting it all together:** Place the prepared chicken over the molokhia stew and pour a spoonful or two of the prepared vinegar-and-onion dressing on top. If serving with pita chips, preheat the oven to 375°F to toast the pita bread, removing it once it is crisp and golden brown. Crumble the toasted pita into a small bowl. Sprinkle the desired amount of toasted pita chips over each portion.

May be served as is or with rice. If serving with rice, add rice to each plate first, followed by the molokhia stew and chicken. Top with the vinegar-and-onion dressing.

Cook's secret: Roast the onions and garlic prior to combining with the molokhia.

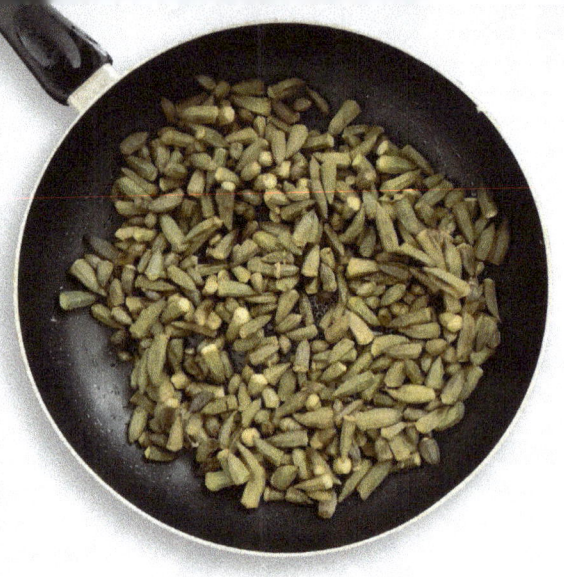

OKRA AND MEAT STEW WITH RICE

(BAMIA BI LAHM MA RIZ)

Serves 4–6
Total time (preparation & cooking): 2 hours, 10 minutes

---

nutritional information per serving (22.4 oz.) — **Cal** 646 **Fat** 27.9g (sat 9g) **Chol** 92mg **Carbs** 67g **Sugars** 4g **Protein** 34g **Fiber** 8g **Sodium** 969mg **Vit. A** (48% DV) **Vit. C** (83% DV) **Calcium** (19% DV) **Iron** (23% DV)

INGREDIENTS

- 1 tablespoon salted butter
- 4 tablespoons extra-virgin olive oil
- 2 pounds fresh okra (with stems removed)
- 1 large lemon, freshly squeezed
- 1½ pounds lamb shanks (may substitute with sirloin cubes)
- 1 teaspoon table salt
- ½ teaspoon black pepper, coarsely ground
- 1 teaspoon cinnamon powder
- ½ teaspoon allspice, ground
- 10 garlic cloves, peeled and halved
- 2 large tomatoes, diced
- 1 bunch fresh cilantro, chopped (about 2 cups)
- 1 teaspoon tomato paste
- 1 pinch of cayenne (optional)
- 2½ cups water

Vermicelli rice

- 2 cups medium-grain Egyptian white rice (may substitute with Arborio rice)
- 2 tablespoons sunflower oil
- ¾ stick salted butter (3 ounces)
- 2 cups vermicelli (egg noodles)
- 2½ cups water
- 1 teaspoon table salt

INSTRUCTIONS

1. **Preparing the okra:** In a large frying pan, heat the butter and 1 tablespoon of the olive oil. Add the okra and sauté for 8 to 10 minutes. Add the lemon and turn off the heat. Set aside.

2. **Preparing the lamb stew:** In a large stockpot or rondeau with about a six-quart capacity, heat the remaining 3 tablespoons of olive oil. Add the lamb shanks, table salt, black pepper, cinnamon powder, and allspice. Stir and cook on low heat for 15 minutes. Add the garlic cloves and cook for several more minutes. Stir in the tomatoes and fresh cilantro. Continue to cook on low heat for about 5 more minutes. Then add the tomato paste, the cayenne (if desired), and the water. Bring to a boil. Lower heat and cook for 1 hour and 10 minutes, or until the lamb is tender and flakes off the bone. Check the stew to make sure there is sufficient broth or stock, adding water if needed. Add the okra and cook for another 25 to 30 minutes.

3. **Preparing the vermicelli rice:** Rinse the rice, drain, and set aside. In a medium saucepan, heat the sunflower oil and ½ stick of the butter. Add the vermicelli and stir. Once the vermicelli turns golden brown, add the water, rice, table salt, and the remaining ¼ stick of butter. Bring to a boil and reduce heat to low. Cook covered on low heat for 20 to 25 minutes, or until the rice is cooked. Turn off but do not remove from the heat. Cover with a towel and allow to sit 10 minutes before serving.

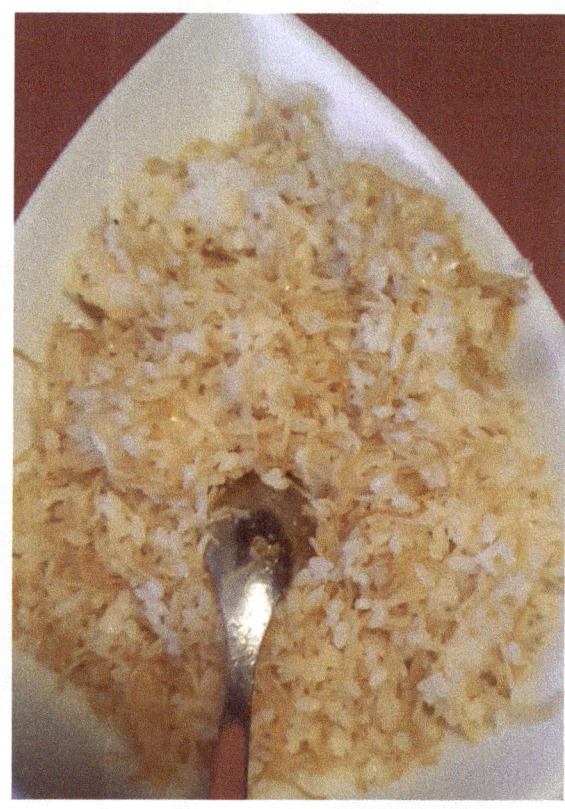

May serve the okra and rice separately or with the okra over the rice.

Cook's secret: Sauté the okra, and finish off with squeezed lemon.

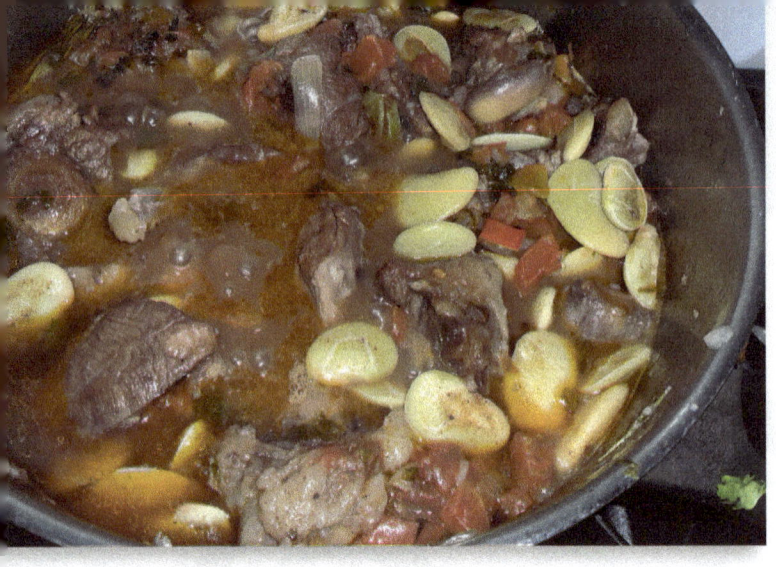

LIMA BEANS AND MEAT STEW
(FASOLIA BI LAHM)

Serves 4–6
Total time (preparation & cooking):
2 hours, 45 minutes + 12 hours soaking

---

nutritional information per serving (18.5 oz.)

Cal 430 **Fat** 13.2g (sat 3.3g) **Chol** 116mg **Carbs** 28g **Sugars** 6g **Protein** 51g **Fiber** 7g **Sodium** 1392mg **Vit. A** (21% DV) **Vit. C** (41% DV) **Calcium** (10% DV) **Iron** (29% DV)

INGREDIENTS

1	pound dried lima beans (may substitute with dried navy beans or fresh shell October beans)
9	cups water
3	tablespoons extra-virgin olive oil
2	large onions, medium-diced
5	peeled garlic cloves, cut in half
2	pounds sirloin steak, cut in cubes (may substitute with lamb shanks)
1	tablespoon tomato paste
2	teaspoons table salt
2	teaspoons cinnamon powder
1½	teaspoons allspice, ground
½	teaspoon cayenne (optional)
3	medium tomatoes, diced
1	bunch fresh cilantro, chopped (about 2 cups)
¼	cup lemon juice (freshly squeezed or bottled)

INSTRUCTIONS

1. **Preparing the beans:** Rinse the lima beans with water before soaking. Place the lima beans in a large bowl with enough water to cover the beans. Allow the lima beans to soak overnight for about 12 hours. When complete, strain the lima beans and discard the soak water. Rinse the lima beans well using a colander. In a large saucepan, bring 5 cups of the water to a low boil and add the lima beans. Boil for 15 minutes uncovered on medium heat. Strain the lima beans and set aside. (If using fresh shell October beans, do not soak overnight or boil—they are ready to use after removing from pods.)

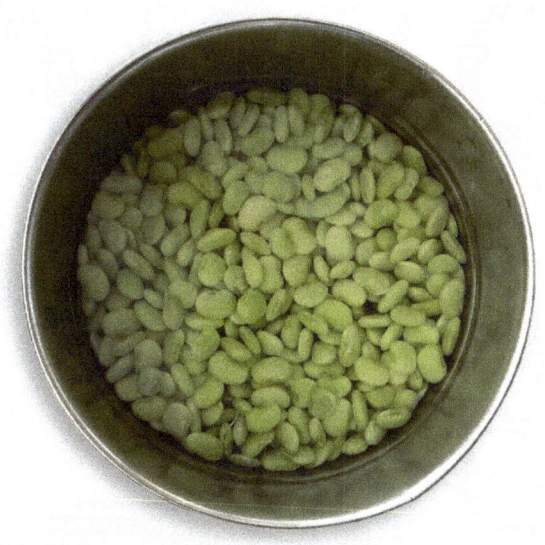

2. **Preparing the meat stew and adding the beans:** In a large stockpot or rondeau with six-quart capacity, heat the olive oil and onions together. After a few minutes, stir in the garlic cloves and sirloin cubes. Continue frying uncovered until the meat is lightly browned. Add the tomato paste, table salt, cinnamon powder, allspice, and cayenne (if desired). Slowly stir in the tomatoes and cilantro. Add the prepared lima beans and lemon juice. Cook covered for 20 minutes on low heat, stirring gently. Remove lid and add the remaining 4 cups of water. Bring to a boil and reduce heat to low. Cook for another 1 hour and 30 minutes to 1 hour 45 minutes covered. Add more water as needed to prevent the beans from sticking to the pot.

May be served as is or with vermicelli rice.

Cook's secret: Boil the beans after soaking, and use fresh cilantro in the meat sauce.

PEA STEW AND RICE
(YAKHNI BI BAZELLA MA RIZ)

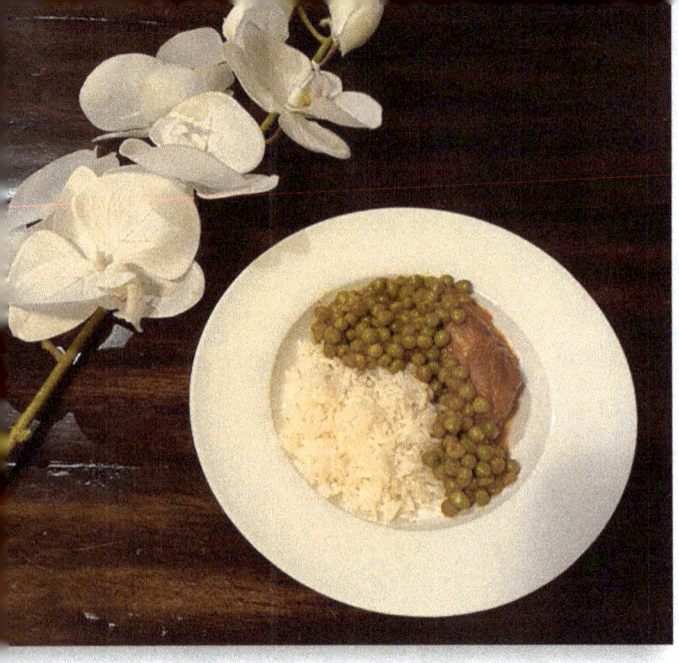

Serves 4–6
Total time (preparation & cooking):
2 hours, 35 minutes

nutritional information per serving (18.9 oz.)	Cal 500 Fat 19.2g (sat 5.8g) Chol 58mg Carbs 57g Sugars 16g Protein 26g Fiber 10g Sodium 889mg Vit. A (32% DV) Vit. C (103% DV) Calcium (10% DV) Iron (28% DV)

INGREDIENTS

- 2 tablespoons sunflower oil
- 1 large onion, medium-diced
- 6 garlic cloves, peeled and chopped
- 1 pound lamb shanks (may substitute with sirloin cubes)
- ¾ teaspoon allspice, ground
- 1 teaspoon cinnamon powder
- 1 tablespoon black pepper, coarsely ground
- ½ teaspoon cayenne (optional)
- 2 large tomatoes, diced
- 1 teaspoon sea salt
- 2½ cups water
- 1 teaspoon tomato paste
- 1 tablespoon pomegranate molasses
- 1½ pounds green peas, thawed if frozen
- 1 (6-ounce) jar of whole artichoke hearts (optional)

RICE

- 1 cup white basmati rice
- 1½ cups water
- ½ stick salted butter (2 ounces)
- 1 teaspoon sea salt
- 2 tablespoons extra-virgin olive oil

INSTRUCTIONS

1. **Preparing the lamb and pea stew:** Heat the sunflower oil on low in a large stockpot or rondeau with about a five-quart capacity. Add the onions and sauté for 3 to 4 minutes. Add the garlic cloves and continue to sauté on low heat for an additional minute or two. Stir in the lamb shanks, allspice, cinnamon powder, black pepper, and cayenne if desired. Cook the lamb shanks for about 10 minutes, or until evenly browned. Stir in the tomatoes and sea salt. Combine the water with the tomato paste, and add to the stew. Stir to combine. Add the pomegranate molasses. Stir in the peas and cook over medium-low heat for 1 hour, or until lamb is flaky and tender. If desired, add artichoke hearts to the stew, making sure to drain them beforehand to remove the brine. Cook the stew for another 20 minutes on low-medium heat.

2. **Preparing the rice:** Rinse the rice, drain, and set aside. In a saucepan, bring the water to a boil. Add the rice and reduce heat to low. Add the butter, sea salt, and olive oil. Cover the rice and cook for 15 to 20 minutes. Turn off the heat and place a kitchen towel over the saucepan, allowing the rice to sit for 10 minutes before serving.

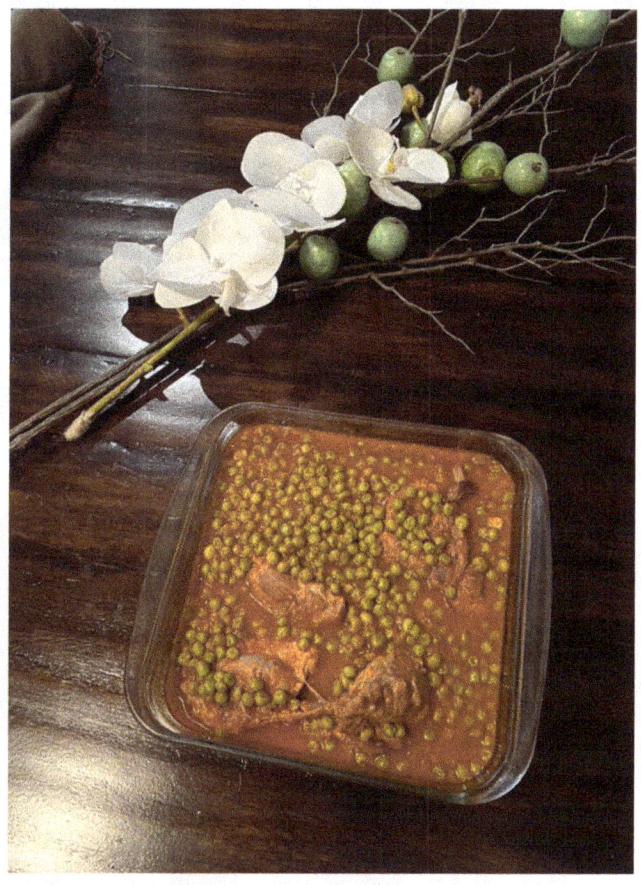

May serve the stew and rice separately or with the stew over the rice.

Cook's secret: Use lamb shanks in the stew.

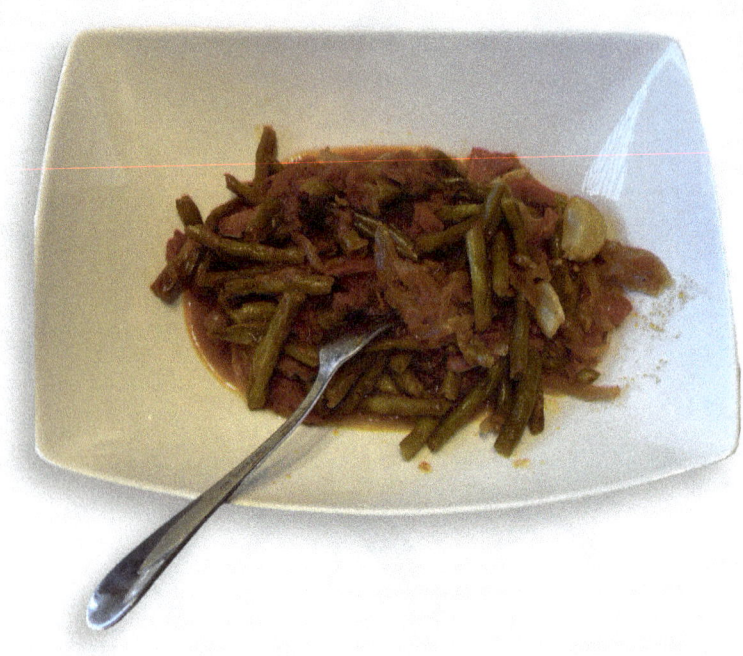

GREEN BEAN STEW
(LOUBIEH BI ZAYT)

Serves 4
Total time (preparation & cooking):
1 hour, 40 minutes

---

nutritional information per serving (14.9 oz.) — **Cal** 212 **Fat** 10.8g (sat 1.5g) **Chol** 0mg **Carbs** 28g **Sugars** 15g **Protein** 5g **Fiber** 7g **Sodium** 824mg **Vit. A** (76% DV) **Vit. C** (81% DV) **Calcium** (11% DV) **Iron** (15% DV)

INGREDIENTS

- 1 pound fresh green beans, preferably romano beans or french beans (may substitute with frozen green beans, thawed)
- 3 tablespoons extra-virgin olive oil
- 2 medium sweet onions, cut into thin strips
- 7 garlic cloves, peeled and halved
- 2 large tomatoes, diced
- 1 teaspoon table salt
- 1 small, fresh hot chili pepper, finely chopped with seeds removed (may substitute with ¼ teaspoon cayenne)
- ½ teaspoon black pepper, coarsely ground
- ½ cup water
- 1 teaspoon tomato paste
- 1 tablespoon dried mint

INSTRUCTIONS

1. **Preparing the green beans:** Using a colander, rinse the fresh green beans in cool water and drain well. Break off both ends at the tips and pull to remove any string. Set aside.

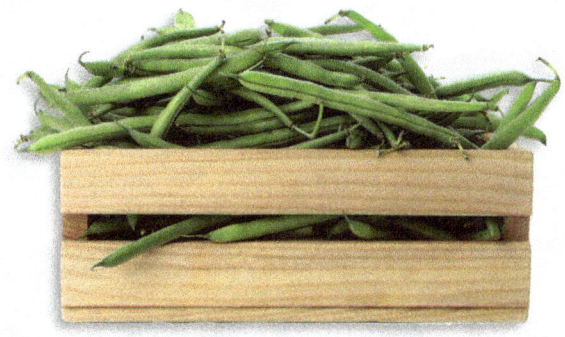

2. **Preparing the onions and garlic:** Heat the olive oil on low in a large skillet. Add the onions and sauté for 3 to 4 minutes, or until they begin to change color. Add the garlic and continue to sauté for a few minutes, or until the cloves turn light golden brown.

3. **Putting the green bean stew together:** Fold the prepared green beans into the skillet with the prepared onions and garlic. Then add the tomatoes, table salt, chili pepper, and black pepper. Cook for 15 minutes on low heat. Stir in the water and tomato paste. Cover and continue to cook on low for another 30 minutes. Empty contents onto a serving plate and sprinkle the dried mint on top. Serve warm or chilled.

May be served as is or with pita bread.

Cook's secret: Sauté the onions and garlic before adding the green beans.

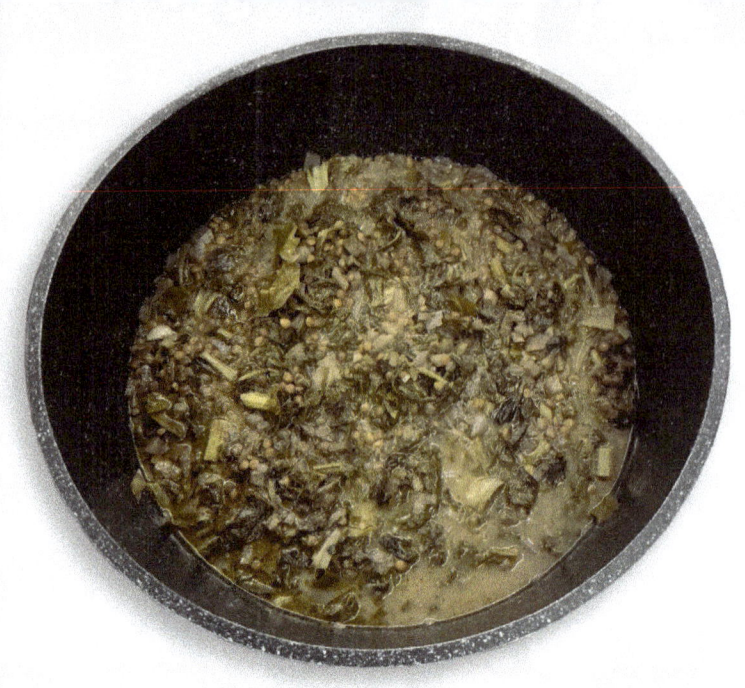

LENTIL STEW WITH SWISS CHARD AND LEMON

(ADAS BI HAMOUD)

Serves 4–6
Total time (preparation & cooking):
3 hours, 20 minutes

nutritional information per serving (21.5 oz.)	**Cal** 443 **Fat** 33g (sat 4.6g) **Chol** 0mg **Carbs** 32g **Sugars** 6g **Protein** 8g **Fiber** 8g **Sodium** 417mg **Vit. A** (190% DV) **Vit. C** (64% DV) **Calcium** (11% DV) **Iron** (23% DV)

INGREDIENTS

- ¾ cup extra-virgin olive oil
- 1 large onion, chopped
- 4 garlic cloves, peeled and minced
- 1 garlic clove, peeled and mashed
- 1 medium russet potato, peeled and diced
- 1 medium sweet potato, peeled and diced
- 2½ tablespoons sumac
- 7 cups water
- ½ teaspoon table salt
- 1½ cups brown lentils, rinsed and drained
- 8 stalks Swiss chard, coarsely chopped
- ¼ cup lemon juice (freshly squeezed or bottled)
- ¼ teaspoon black pepper, coarsely ground
- ¼ teaspoon cayenne
- ½ teaspoon cumin, ground
- ½ teaspoon allspice, ground

INSTRUCTIONS

1. **Preparing the potatoes:** In a medium saucepan, add the olive oil, onion, and minced and mashed garlic. Cook on medium heat until the onion is translucent and light brown. Add the russet potatoes and sweet potatoes and reduce heat to low. Cook for 20 minutes, stirring occasionally. Add 1 tablespoon of the sumac and cook for another 5 minutes on low heat. Set aside.

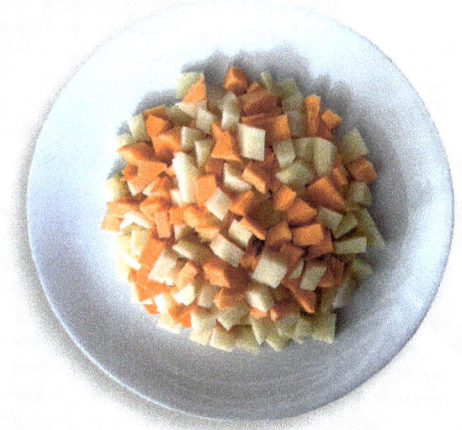

2. **Preparing the lentil stew and adding the potatoes:** In a large stockpot or rondeau with about a five-quart capacity, bring the water to a boil and add the table salt. Reduce heat to medium and add the lentils. Cover the pot and cook on medium heat for 1 hour and 15 minutes, or until lentils are tender. Check periodically during cooking to ensure that water quantity is sufficient. Add water if the stew is too thick. Stir in the Swiss chard and lemon juice. Slowly add the prepared russet and sweet potatoes to the stockpot. Add the black pepper, cayenne, cumin, allspice, and the remaining 1½ tablespoons of sumac. Reduce heat to low. Cook the stew for an additional 35 to 45 minutes, stirring occasionally. Serve hot or warm.

Best served as is.

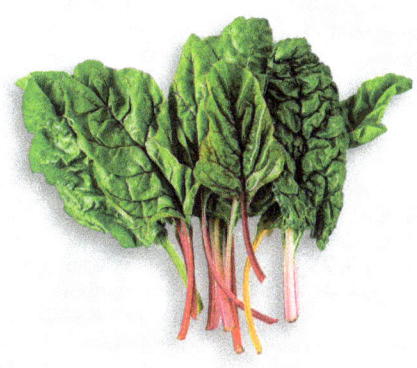

Cook's secret: Use both sumac and lemon for tangy flavor.

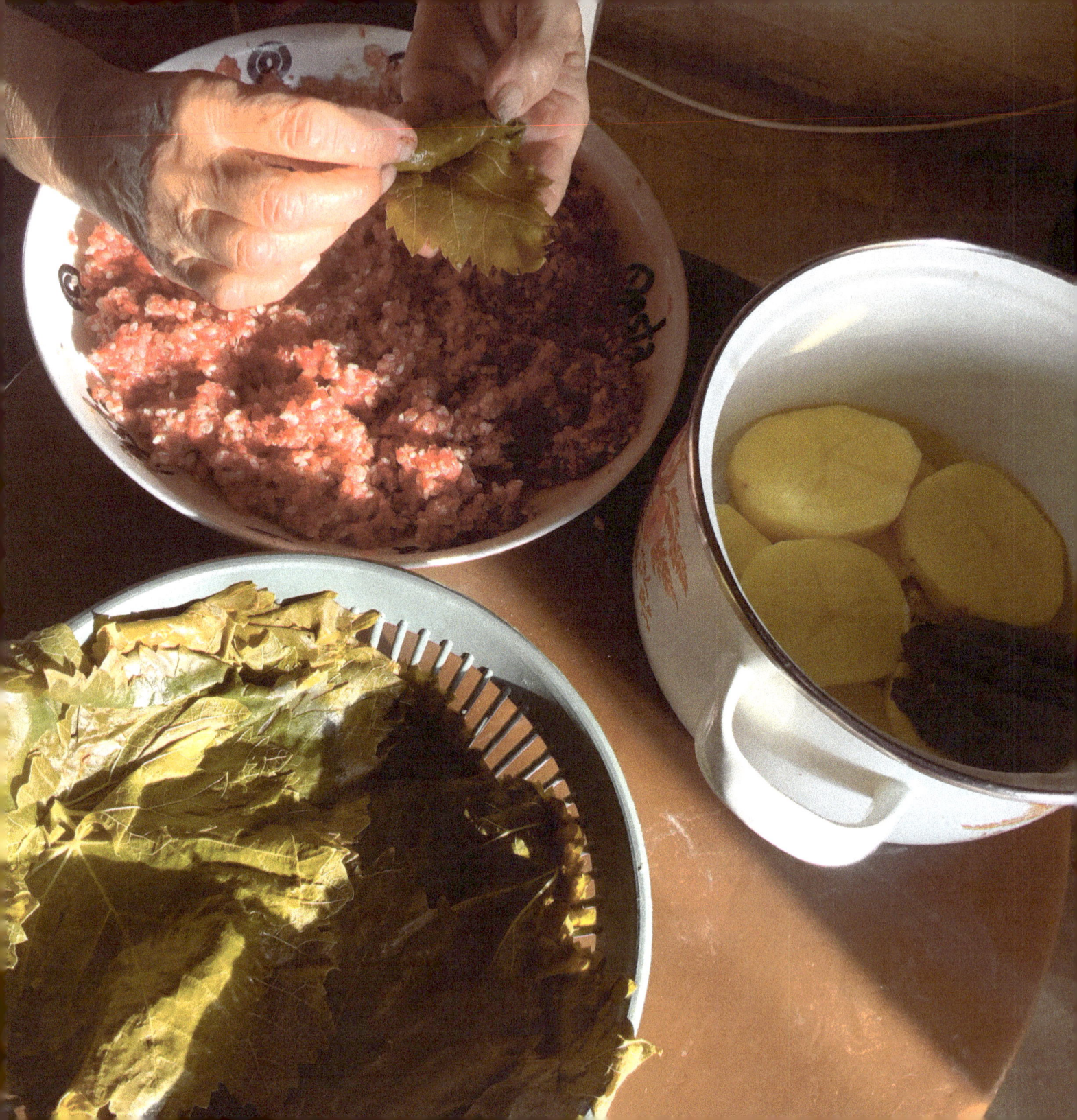

Stuffed Vegetables & Vines

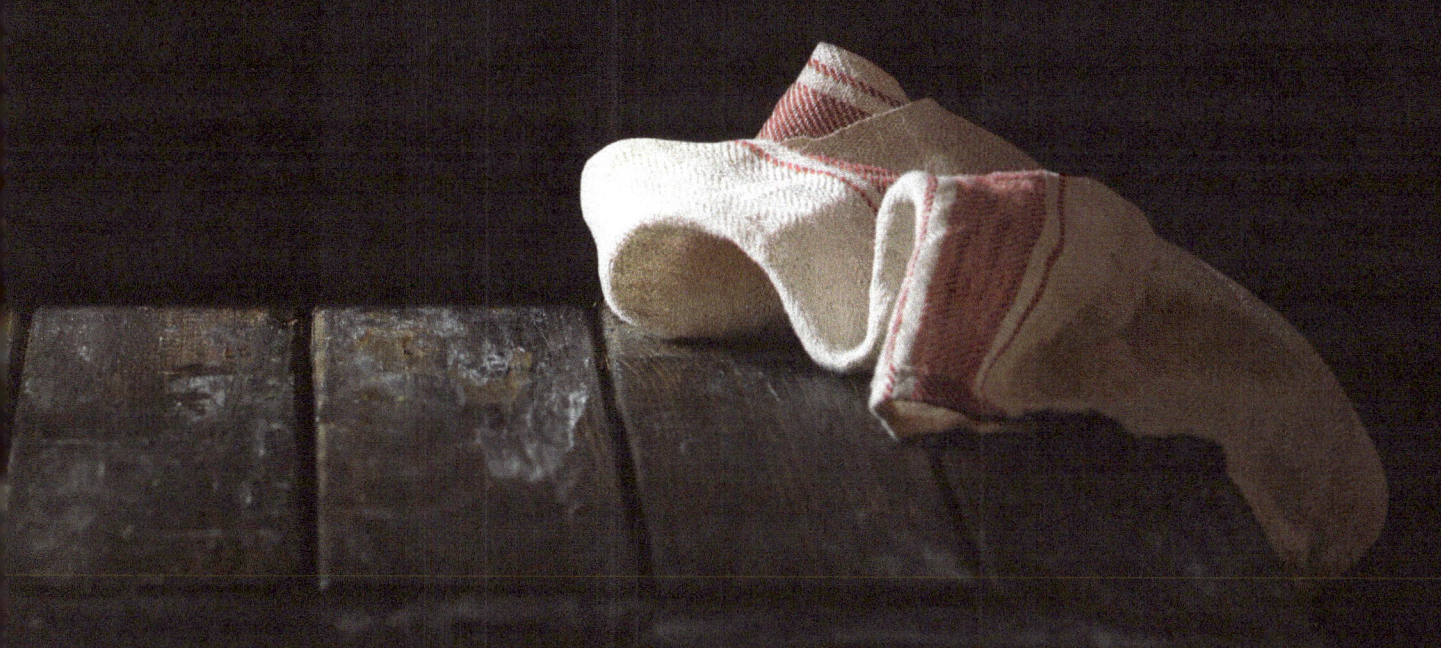

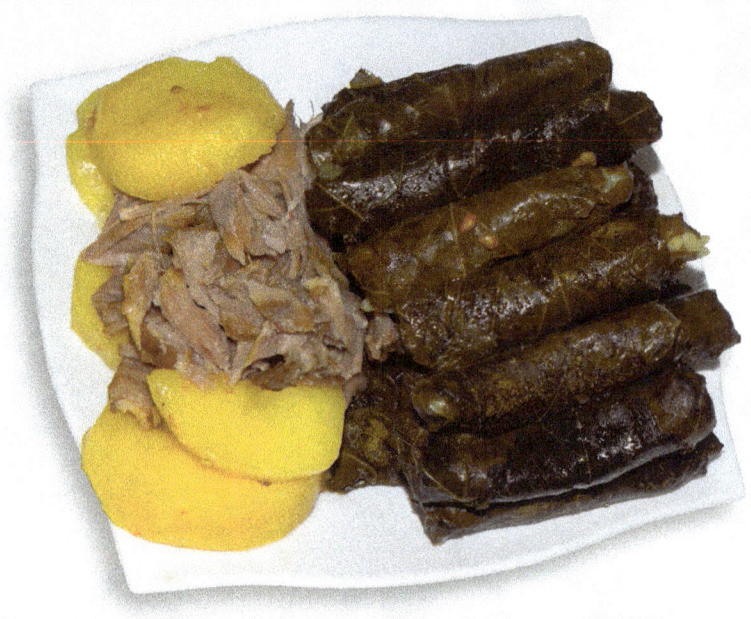

STUFFED GRAPE LEAVES WITH MEAT
(WARAK ENAB BI LAHM)

Serves 6–8
Total time (preparation & cooking):
3 hours, 30 minutes

---

nutritional information per serving (13.1 oz.) — **Cal** 676 **Fat** 44.7g (sat 16.2g) **Chol** 111mg **Carbs** 39g **Sugars** 4g **Protein** 32g **Fiber** 8g **Sodium** 428mg **Vit. A** (316% DV) **Vit. C** (21% DV) **Calcium** (25% DV) **Iron** (24% DV)

INGREDIENTS

- 1 pound (16-ounce) jar grape leaves
- 1 cup medium-grain Egyptian white rice (may substitute with Arborio rice)
- 1½ pounds ground lamb (may substitute with ground sirloin)
- 1½ teaspoons allspice, ground
- 1½ teaspoons cinnamon powder
- 1 teaspoon black pepper, coarsely ground
- 4 tablespoons lemon juice (freshly squeezed or bottled)
- 1 teaspoon sea salt
- ½ stick butter (2 ounces), melted
- 6 tablespoons extra-virgin olive oil
- 1 pound lamb rib chops (bone-in)
- 1 russet potato, peeled and sliced into disks ¾ inch thick
- 1 vine-ripe tomato, sliced into disks ½ inch thick
- 5 cardamom, whole
- 2½ cups water

INSTRUCTIONS

1. **Preparing the grape leaves:** Place the grape leaves in a bowl with cold water. Drain and repeat the process three times to remove salt. Set them aside to dry. Remove stems once dried.

2. **Preparing the stuffing:** In a medium-size bowl, combine the rice with the ground meat. Add ½ teaspoon of the allspice, 1 teaspoon of the cinnamon powder, ½ teaspoon of the black pepper, 3½ tablespoons of the lemon juice, and ½ teaspoon of the sea salt. Mix the ingredients by hand. Add the melted butter and 2 tablespoons of the olive oil. Mix again by hand to combine and set aside.

3. **Preparing the lamb chops:** Season the lamb chops with the remaining ½ teaspoon of sea salt, 1 teaspoon of allspice, ½ teaspoon of black pepper, and ½ teaspoon of cinnamon powder. Heat 2 tablespoons of the olive oil in a deep pan and add the lamb chops. Sear the lamb chops on medium heat for 3 to 4 minutes on each side. Add the remaining ½ tablespoon of lemon juice and remove from the heat.

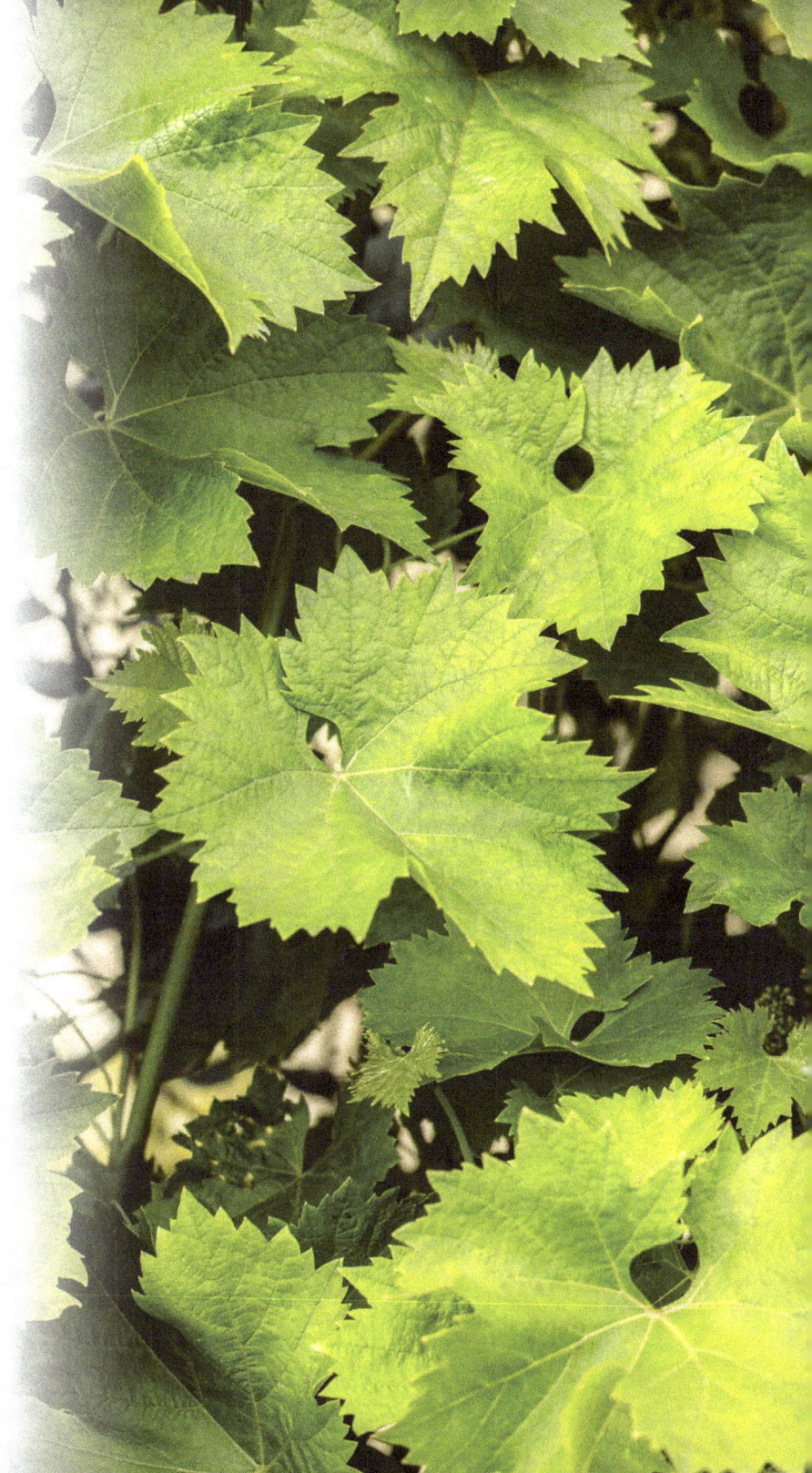

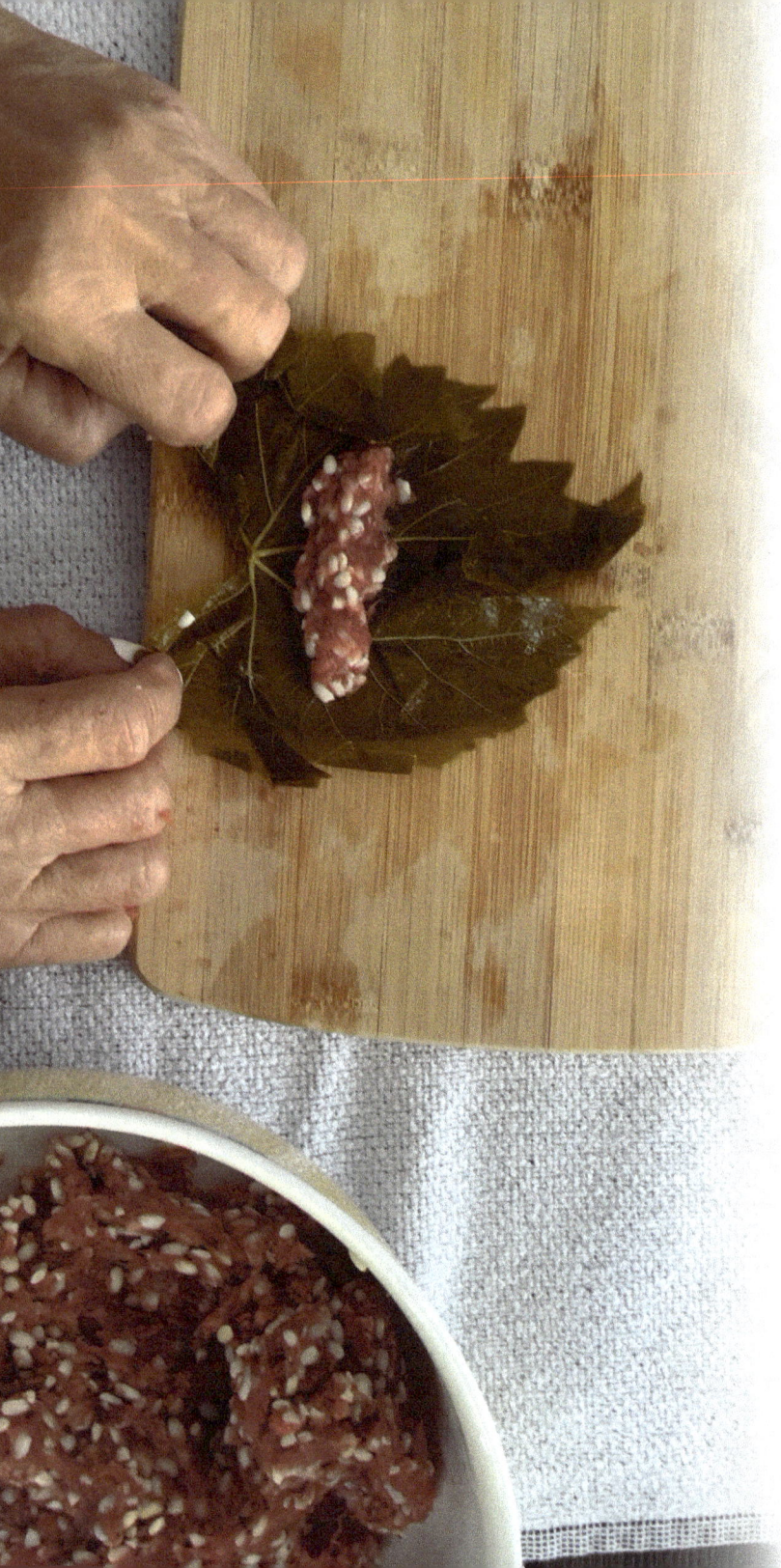

4. **Wrapping the grape leaves and arranging them in the stockpot:** In a large stockpot or rondeau with handles and about a five-quart capacity, add the remaining 2 tablespoons of olive oil. Line the bottom of the stockpot with the sliced potato (peeled) and sliced tomato to provide flavor and prevent sticking while cooking. Next, place half the seared lamb chops over the potato and tomato. Start wrapping and arranging the grape leaves on top of the lamb chops.

To wrap the grape leaves, place each leaf vein side up on a large plate. Drop about 1 heaping tablespoon of the prepared stuffing onto each grape leaf, spreading it into a thin line. Make sure to leave enough room on both sides for rolling, folding the sides inward to roll. Place the rolled grape leaf in the pot. Repeat and arrange the stuffed grape leaves tightly side by side in the pot with no gaps. Continue by adding another layer of grape leaves, until all the leaves are used.

5. **Cooking the grape leaves:** Once the stockpot is lined with its final layer of grape leaves, arrange the rest of the prepared lamb chops on top of the grape leaves. Place a small plate facedown over the lamb chops and grape leaves to prevent the grape leaves from opening and moving during cooking. Add the cardamom and the water. When adding water, adjust the quantity so that the water level is just below the small plate. Do not remove the plate during cooking. Bring to a boil on medium-high heat and then immediately reduce heat to low. Simmer covered for 2 hours and 30 minutes on low heat. Cooking time and water quantity can be adjusted as needed.

When the grape leaves are finished cooking and the rice is tender, remove from the heat and allow to cool (covered) for at least 25 minutes before serving. To transfer to a serving plate, remove the lid from the stockpot and take out the small plate. If needed, drain any excess (unabsorbed) liquid from the pot to avoid spillage during transfer. Place a shallow serving plate that is a little larger than the stockpot facedown over the pot. Using oven mitts or pot holders, grip the plate firmly over the pot handles. Once grip is secure, flip the pot upside down in one swift motion so that the plate ends up on the bottom and the grape leaves covered with sliced potato and tomato end up on top. Gently lower the plate onto a counter surface and then lift up to remove the stockpot.

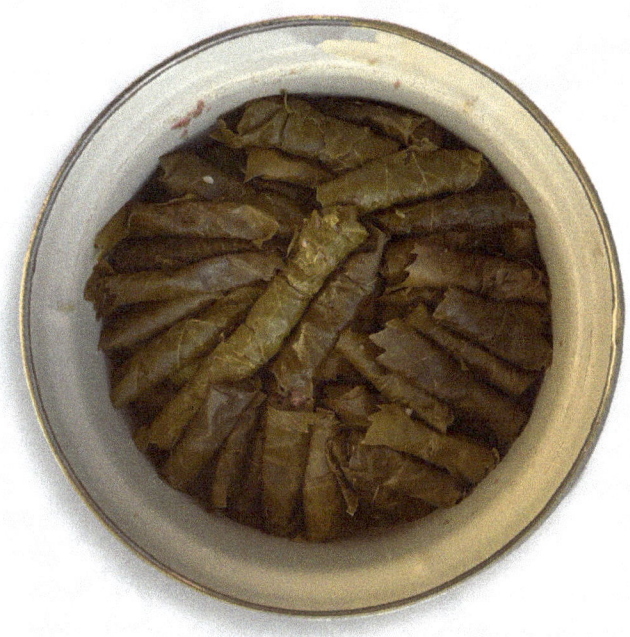

Best served as is.

Cook's secret: Sear the lamb chops, and then cook them with the grape leaves.

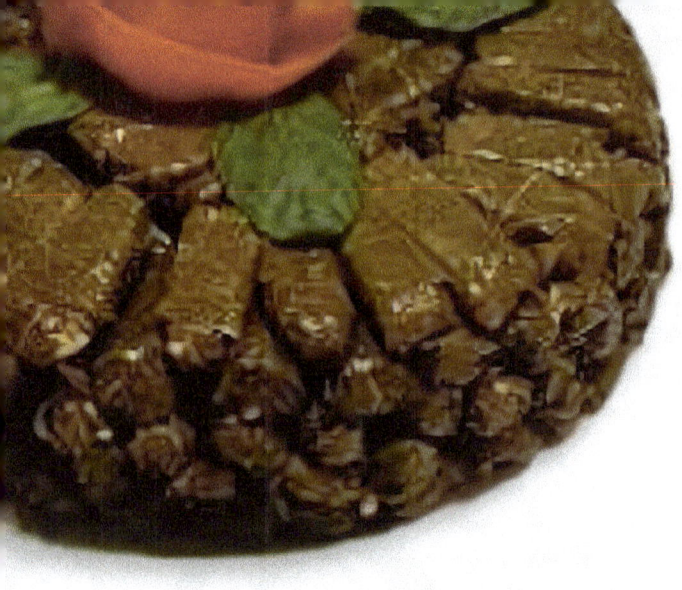

STUFFED GRAPE LEAVES WITHOUT MEAT

(WARAK ENAB BI ZAYT)

Serves 4–6
Total time (preparation & cooking):
3 hours, 30 minutes

---

nutritional information per serving (11.6 oz.) — **Cal** 383 **Fat** 15.9g (sat 2.7g) **Chol** 19mg **Carbs** 50g **Sugars** 8g **Protein** 14g **Fiber** 10g **Sodium** 537mg **Vit. A** (389% DV) **Vit. C** (98% DV) **Calcium** (30% DV) **Iron** (23% DV)

INGREDIENTS

- 1 pound (16-ounce) jar grape leaves
- 2 bunches Italian flat parsley, finely chopped
- 1 bunch fresh mint, finely chopped
- 1 cup medium-grain Egyptian white rice (may substitute with Arborio rice)
- 4 vine-ripe tomatoes, finely chopped
- 1 fresh hot pepper, finely chopped with seeds removed
- ½ teaspoon black pepper, coarsely ground
- 1½ teaspoons sea salt
- 2 lemons, freshly squeezed
- 6 tablespoons extra-virgin olive oil
- 1 russet potato, peeled and sliced into disks ¾ inch thick
- 1 vine-ripe tomato, sliced into disks ½ inch thick
- 1 large sweet onion, sliced into disks ½ inch thick
- 7 garlic cloves, peeled and diced
- 1½ cups water

INSTRUCTIONS

1. **Preparing the grape leaves:** Place the grape leaves in a bowl with cold water. Drain and repeat the process three times to remove salt. Set them aside to dry. Remove stems once dried.

2. **Preparing the vegetarian stuffing:** Place the parsley (without stems) and mint in a medium bowl. Fill the bowl with water. Drain using a fine mesh sieve. Repeat this process several times to remove all the dirt. Set aside. Rinse the rice with cool water and drain. In a separate medium bowl, combine the drained rice with the drained parsley and mint. Add the tomatoes, hot pepper, black pepper, and 1 teaspoon of the sea salt. Mix to combine. Add 1 squeezed lemon and 5 tablespoons of the olive oil. Mix again to thoroughly combine and set aside.

3. **Wrapping the grape leaves and arranging them in the stockpot:** In a large stockpot or rondeau with handles and about a five-quart capacity, add the remaining 1 tablespoon of olive oil. Line the bottom of the stockpot with the sliced potato (peeled), tomato, and onion to provide flavor and prevent sticking while cooking. Start wrapping the grape leaves. To wrap the grape leaves, place each leaf vein side up on a large plate. Using your hand, remove about 1 tablespoon of the prepared vegetarian stuffing, squeezing it gently to remove excess juices before spreading it into a thin line on each grape leaf. The juices from the stuffing should be saved in the bowl for later cooking. Make sure to leave enough room on both sides of the leaf for rolling, folding the leaves inward to roll.

Place the rolled grape leaf in the pot (on top of the potato, tomato, and onion). Repeat and arrange the stuffed grape leaves tightly side by side and in layered stacks. Sandwich the garlic cloves between the different layers of grape leaves. Continue by adding another layer until all the grape leaves are used.

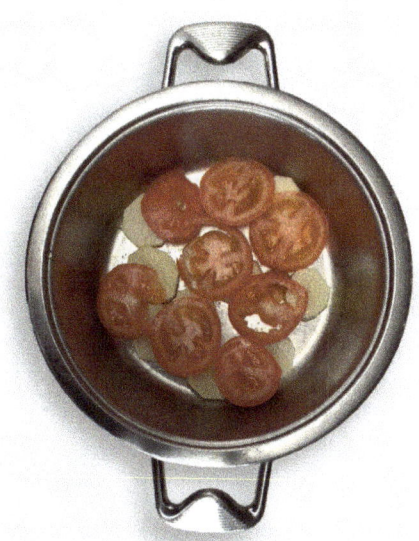

4. **Cooking the grape leaves:** Once the stockpot is lined with its final layer of grape leaves, pour the leftover juices from the vegetable stuffing over the top layer. Add the remaining ½ teaspoon of sea salt and 1 squeezed lemon to the pot. Place a small plate facedown over the grape leaves to prevent them from opening and moving during cooking. Add water, adjusting the quantity if needed so that the water level is just below the plate. Do not remove the plate during cooking. Bring to a boil on medium-high heat and then immediately reduce heat to low. Simmer on low for 1 hour and 30 minutes. Cooking time and water quantity can be adjusted as needed.

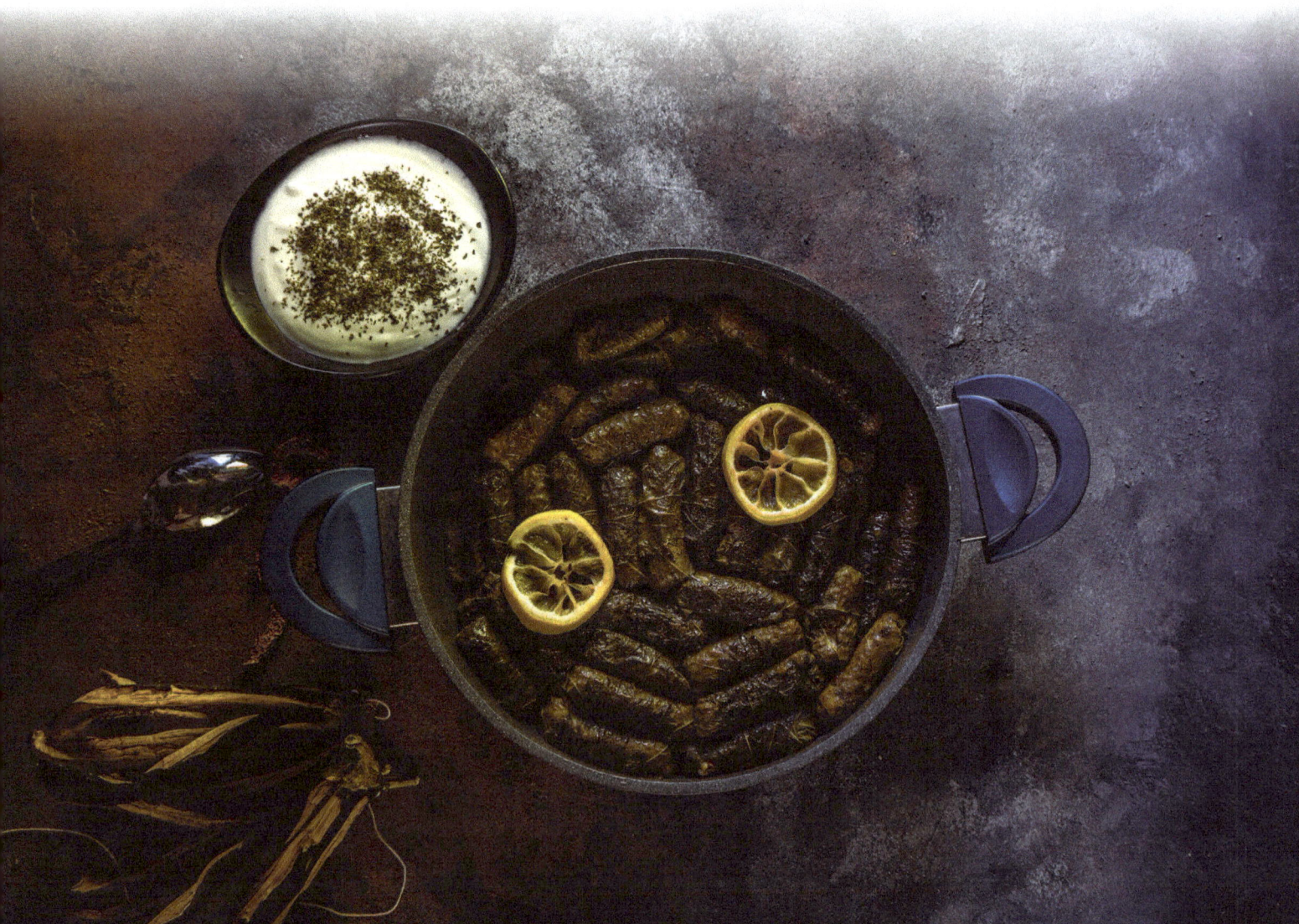

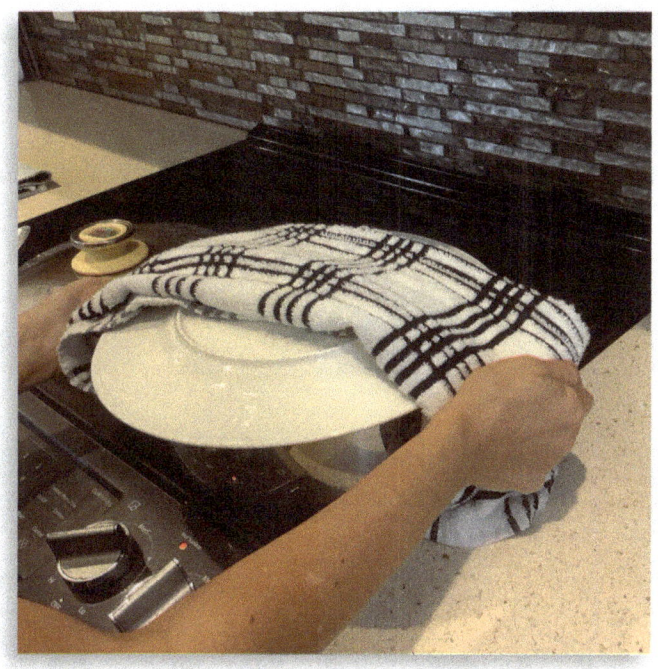 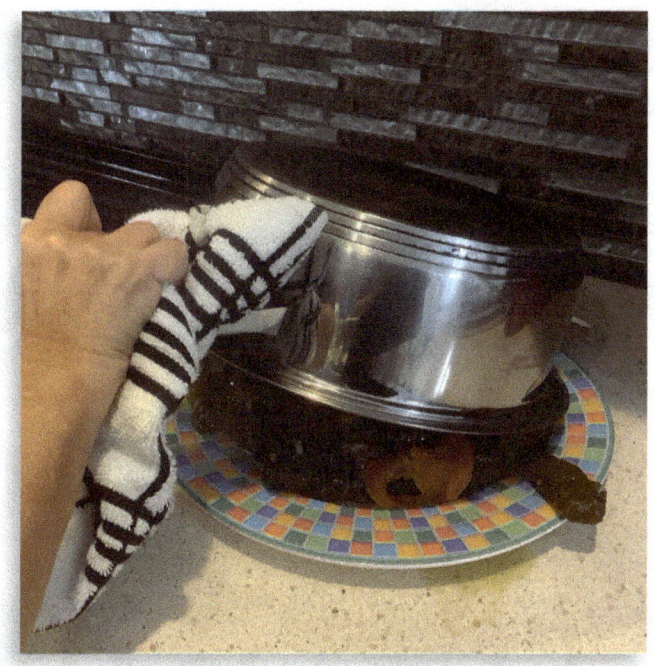

When the grape leaves are finished cooking, remove from the heat and let them cool (covered) for at least 25 minutes. To transfer to a serving plate, remove the lid from the stockpot and take out the small plate. If needed, drain any excess (unabsorbed) liquid from the pot to avoid spillage during transfer. Place a shallow serving plate that is a little larger than the pot facedown over the stockpot. Using oven mitts or pot holders, grip the plate firmly over the pot handles. Once grip is secure, flip the stockpot upside down in one swift motion so that the plate ends up on the bottom and the grape leaves (covered with sliced potato, tomato, and onion) end up on top. Gently lower the plate onto a counter surface and then lift up to remove the stockpot.

Best served as is.

Cook's secret: Use the leftover juices from the stuffing to cook the grape leaves.

STUFFED VEGETABLES & VINES | 39

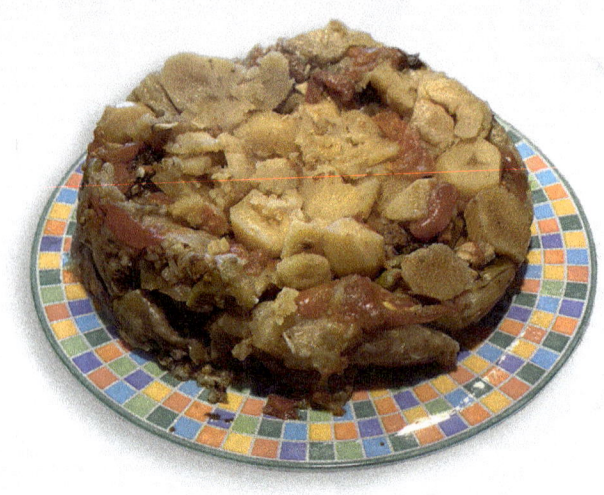

STUFFED CABBAGE ROLLS
(WARAK MALFOUF MAHSHI)

Serves 4–6
Total time (preparation & cooking):
3 hours, 45 minutes

---

nutritional information per serving (9.2 oz.) — **Cal** 567 **Fat** 37.9g (sat 0.9g) **Chol** 116mg **Carbs** 24g **Sugars** 1g **Protein** 37g **Fiber** 5g **Sodium** 499mg **Vit. A** (4% DV) **Vit. C** (26% DV) **Calcium** (9% DV) **Iron** (43% DV)

INGREDIENTS

- 1 teaspoon table salt
- 1 whole green cabbage
- ¾ cup medium-grain Egyptian white rice (may substitute with Arborio rice)
- 1½ pounds ground beef
- 1 teaspoon sea salt
- 1 teaspoon black pepper, coarsely ground
- 1 teaspoon cinnamon powder
- ½ teaspoon allspice, ground
- ½ cup lemon juice (freshly squeezed or bottled)
- 6 tablespoons extra-virgin olive oil
- 2 tomatoes, sliced into disks ½ inch thick
- 1 large russet potato, sliced into disks ¾ inch thick
- 1 pound lamb shoulder chops (bone-in)
- 8 garlic cloves, peeled
- 4 garlic cloves, peeled and mashed
- ¼ cup dried mint

INSTRUCTIONS

1. **Preparing the cabbage:** Fill a large stockpot (with about a six-quart capacity) halfway with water. Bring to a boil and add ½ teaspoon of the table salt. Add the whole head of cabbage core side down and blanch for 10 minutes on medium heat. Rotate or turn the cabbage around in the pot and blanch core side up for 10 minutes, or until the cabbage is tender. Use a pair of thongs or a fork to remove any leaves that come free of the cabbage while boiling. Drain the boiled cabbage into a colander. Allow to cool and peel off cabbage leaves one by one. Cut off the thick parts of the cabbage leaves to prepare for stuffing and rolling. If the center of the cabbage is still hard, return to boiling water for another 3 to 4 minutes, or until cabbage leaves can be easily peeled and removed.

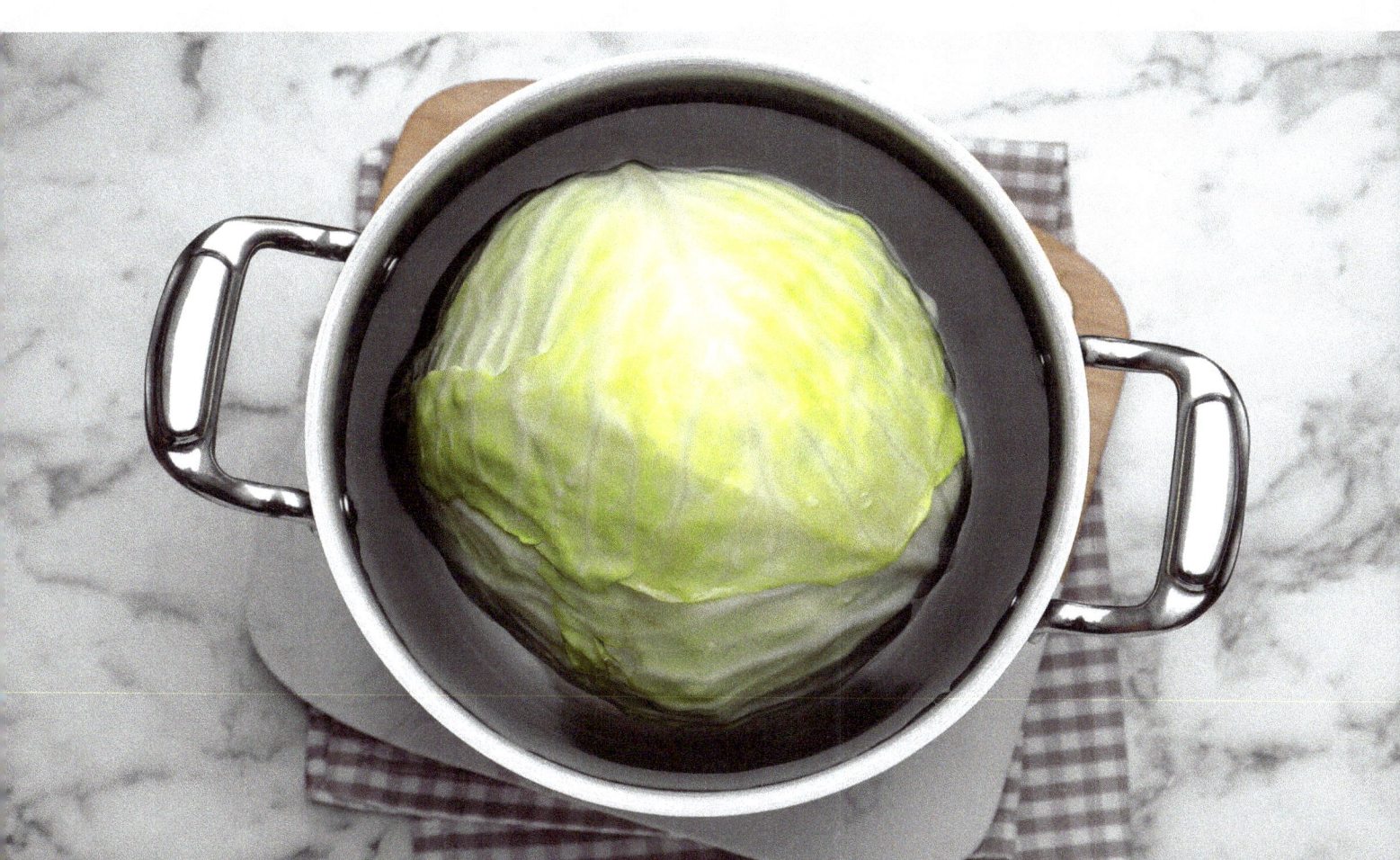

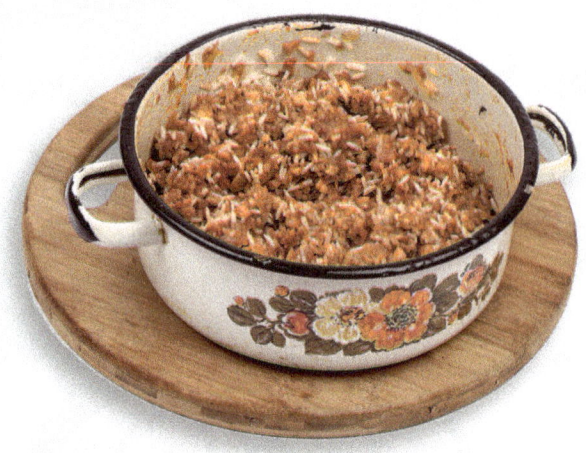

2. **Preparing the rice and beef stuffing:** Soak the rice for 5 minutes in cold water. Drain the rice and mix with the ground beef in a large bowl. Add the sea salt, ½ teaspoon of the black pepper, cinnamon powder, and allspice, along with ¼ cup of the lemon juice and 4 tablespoons of the olive oil. Mix by hand to combine the ingredients.

3. **Stuffing and arranging the cabbage rolls:** Line the sliced tomatoes and potato along the bottom of the large stockpot or rondeau with handles. The stockpot should have about a five-quart capacity. Lay the cabbage leaf flat on a kitchen counter, plate, or cutting board. Fill each cabbage leaf with a spoonful of the rice and beef stuffing. Spread it into a thick line along the edge of the cabbage leaf. Roll and place in the stockpot, vein side down, one by one, on top of the tomatoes and potatoes. Arrange the stuffed cabbage rolls tightly side by side in the pot.

After arranging the first layer of cabbage rolls, prepare the lamb shoulder. Place the lamb shoulder chops on a separate plate and rub both sides with the remaining ½ teaspoon of table salt and ½ teaspoon of black pepper. Once the lamb shoulder chops are evenly seasoned, arrange them over the first or second layer of cabbage rolls. Next, sandwich the garlic cloves between the different layers of cabbage rolls. Continue to layer the stuffed cabbage rolls in stacks until all the stuffing and/or leaves are used.

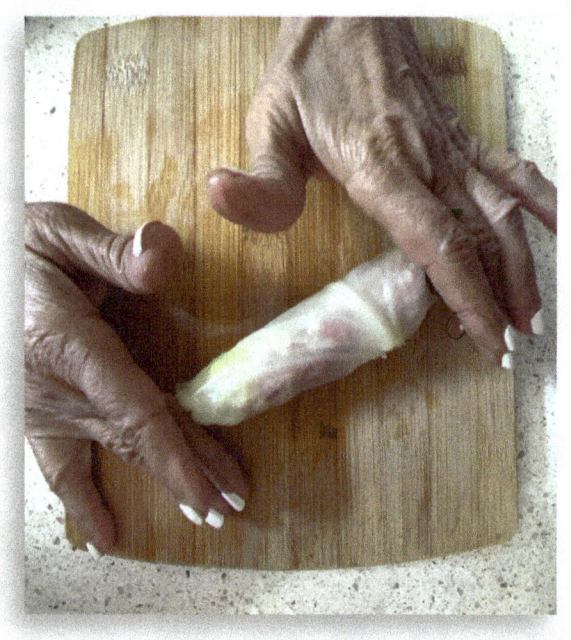

4. **Cooking the cabbage rolls:** In a separate saucepan, fry the mashed garlic with the remaining 2 tablespoons of olive oil for 2 minutes. Pour the entire contents of the saucepan over the cabbage rolls in the stockpot. Add the dried mint and the remaining ¼ cup of lemon juice. Then place a small plate facedown over the cabbage rolls to prevent them from opening and moving during cooking. Gradually add water so that it reaches the top layer of cabbage just below the plate. Bring to a boil and immediately reduce heat to low. Cover and cook for 1 hour and 45 minutes to 2 hours and 15 minutes on low heat. Allow to cool for 25 minutes (covered) before serving.

To transfer to a serving plate, remove the lid from the stockpot and take out the small plate. If needed, drain any excess (unabsorbed) liquid from the pot to avoid spillage during transfer. Place a shallow serving plate that is a little larger than the stockpot facedown over the pot. Using oven mitts or pot holders, grip the plate firmly over the stockpot handles. Once grip is secure, flip the stockpot upside down in one swift motion so that the plate ends up on the bottom and the cabbage rolls covered with tomatoes and potato end up on top. Gently lower the plate onto a counter surface and lift up to remove the pot.

Best served as is.

Cook's secret: Cook the cabbage rolls with lamb shoulder chops.

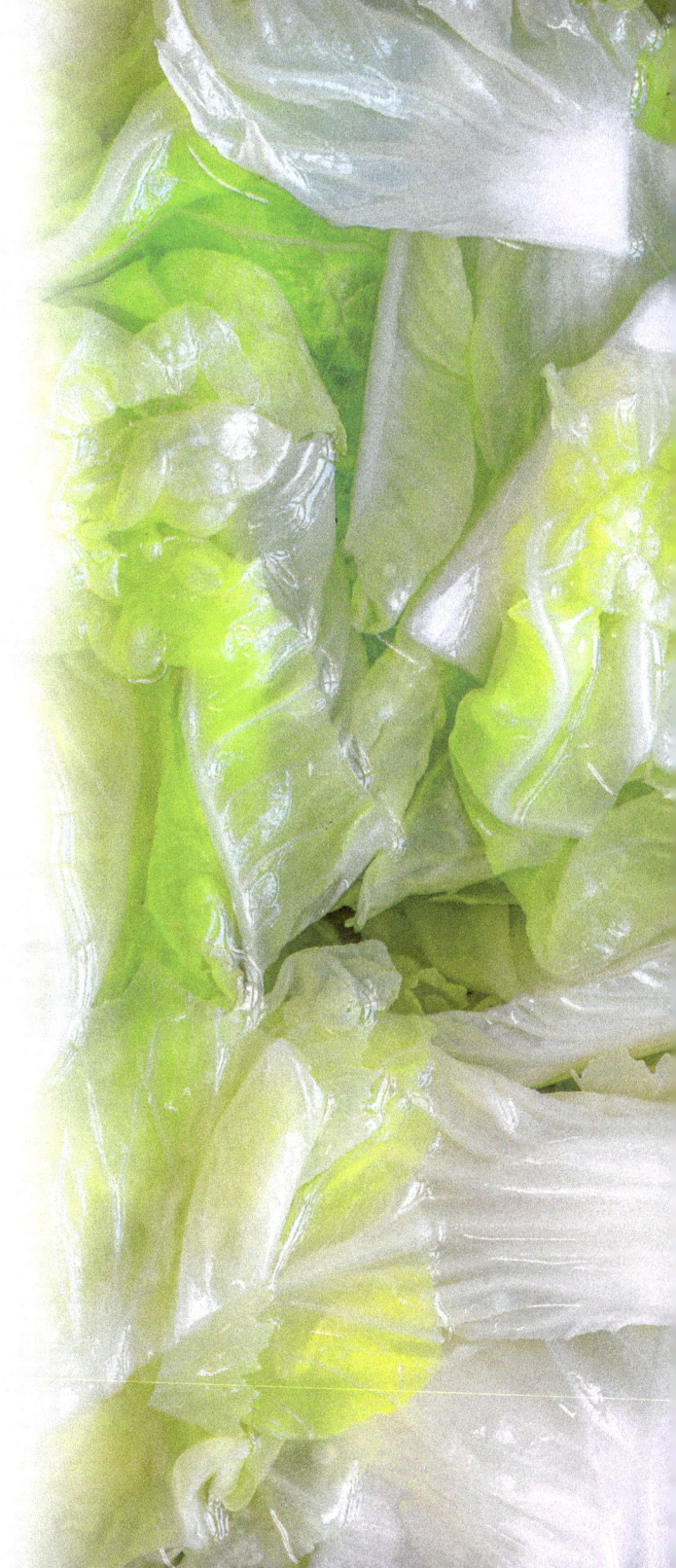

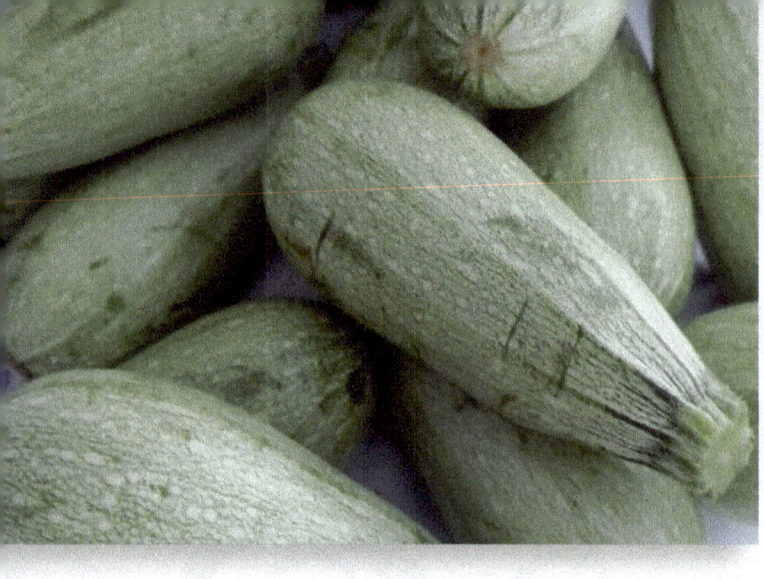

STUFFED COUSA SQUASH

(COUSA MAHSHI)

Serves 4–6
Total time (preparation & cooking):
3 hours, 40 minutes

---

nutritional information per serving (16.9 oz.) — **Cal** 591 **Fat** 30.8g (sat 10.9g) **Chol** 217mg **Carbs** 15g **Sugars** 3g **Protein** 67g **Fiber** 5g **Sodium** 723mg **Vit. A** (26% DV) **Vit. C** (43% DV) **Calcium** (10% DV) **Iron** (41% DV)

INGREDIENTS

- 10 cousa, marrow, or zucchini squash (light green color), cored
- ½ cup medium-grain Egyptian white rice (may substitute with Arborio rice)
- 1½ pounds ground sirloin (may substitute with ground lamb)
- ½ teaspoon allspice, ground
- ½ teaspoon black pepper, coarsely ground
- ¾ teaspoon cinnamon powder
- ¼ teaspoon cayenne
- 1 teaspoon table salt
- 4 tomatoes, medium-diced
- 1½ tablespoons unsalted butter, melted
- 2 tablespoons lemon juice (freshly squeezed or bottled)
- 3 cups water
- 4 pieces of lamb shoulder (about 2 pounds)
- 1 cinnamon stick
- 5 cardamom, whole
- 1 tablespoon tomato paste
- ¼ cup dried mint

Garnish

- 2 tablespoons extra-virgin olive oil
- 1 tablespoon unsalted butter
- 7 garlic cloves, peeled and mashed

INSTRUCTIONS

1. **Preparing the squash:** Wash the squash thoroughly and air-dry, or pat dry with a paper towel. Remove the stems and core the flesh, gently using a corer to avoid puncturing the squash from the inside. Discard the cored flesh.

2. **Preparing the filling and stuffing the squash:** Rinse the rice, drain, and place in a large pan. Then add the ground meat, allspice, black pepper, cinnamon powder, cayenne, table salt, tomatoes, melted butter, and lemon juice to the pan. Mix the ingredients together thoroughly by hand. Stuff each cored squash, making sure to fill to the top without puncturing the squash in the process. Set aside.

3. **Preparing the garlic garnish:** Heat the olive oil and butter in a saucepan on medium heat. Add the garlic cloves, frying until they turn light brown. Remove from the heat and set aside.

4. **Cooking the lamb shoulder and stuffed squash:** In a large stockpot or rondeau with about a six-quart capacity, bring the water to a boil. Reduce heat to low-medium and add the lamb shoulder, cooking for 45 minutes to 1 hour. Add the prepared stuffed squash, cinnamon stick, cardamom, and tomato paste. Stir gently to combine. Cook the squash and lamb together for 45 minutes, checking intermittently to ensure that there is sufficient water. Pour the prepared garlic garnish into the pot over the lamb shoulder and stuffed squash. Add the dried mint and cook for additional 20 to 30 minutes. Serve hot or warm.

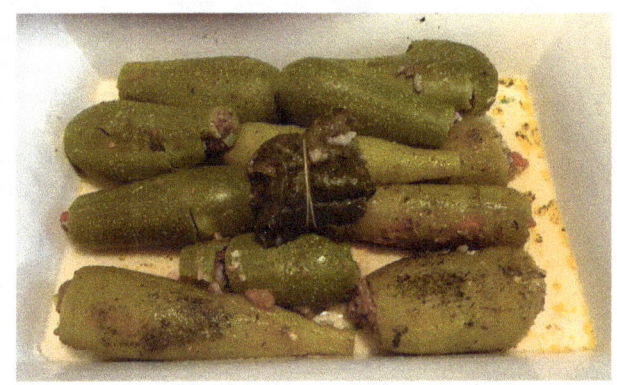

Best served as is.

Cook's secret: Cook the lamb shoulder with the squash.

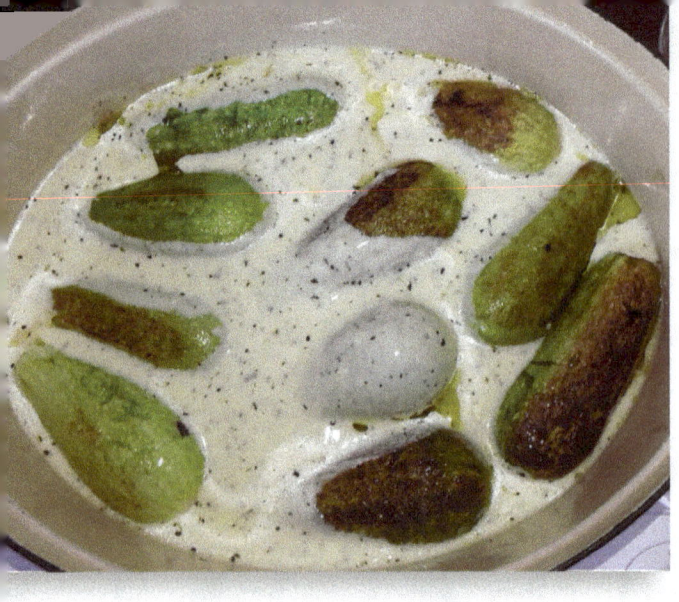

STUFFED COUSA SQUASH WITH YOGHURT SAUCE

(COUSA MAHSHI BI LABAN)

Serves 6
Total time (preparation & cooking):
3 hours, 30 minutes

---

nutritional information per serving (32.4 oz.)

Cal 946 **Fat** 69.9g (sat 21.1g) **Chol** 145mg **Carbs** 43g **Sugars** 25g **Protein** 45g **Fiber** 9g **Sodium** 1004mg **Vit. A** (24% DV) **Vit. C** (150% DV) **Calcium** (30% DV) **Iron** (31% DV)

INGREDIENTS

- 15 cousa, marrow, or zucchini squash (light green color), cored
- 1½ pounds ground lamb (may substitute with ground sirloin)
- 6 tablespoons extra-virgin olive oil
- 2 teaspoons table salt
- 1 teaspoon black pepper, coarsely ground
- 1½ teaspoons cinnamon powder
- 1½ teaspoons allspice, ground
- 1 tablespoon pomegranate molasses
- 2 tablespoons red wine
- ¾ cup pine nuts, whole
- 2 cups sunflower oil
- 4½ cups water
- 6 lamb chops (rib chops preferred)
- 4 garlic, peeled and mashed
- 1 tablespoon unsalted butter
- 5 tablespoons cornstarch
- 2 pounds plain low fat or whole milk yoghurt

46 | LITTLE RECIPE BOOK

INSTRUCTIONS

1. **Preparing the squash:** Wash the squash thoroughly and air-dry, or pat dry with a paper towel. Remove stems and core the flesh gently using a corer to avoid puncturing the squash from the inside. Discard the cored flesh.

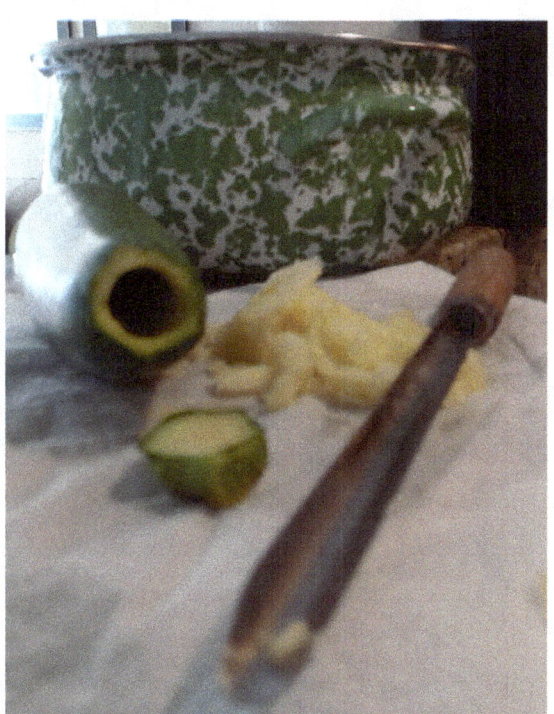

2. **Preparing the squash filling:** In a large, deep saucepan, add the ground meat and 2½ tablespoons of the olive oil. Cook on medium heat, stirring in 1 teaspoon of the table salt, ½ teaspoon of the black pepper, 1 teaspoon of the cinnamon powder, and 1 teaspoon of the allspice. Use a wooden spoon to break up the clumps of meat and evenly spread the spices. Add the pomegranate molasses and continue stirring for another 4 minutes. Add the red wine and stir in ¼ cup of the pine nuts. Cook for an additional 2 minutes and set aside.

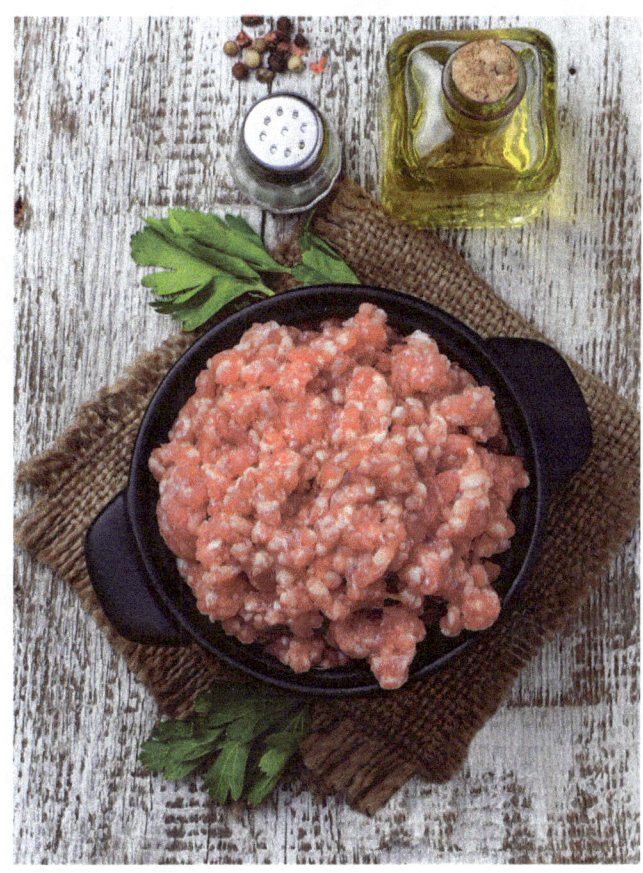

3. **Stuffing and frying the squash:** Generously stuff each cored squash with the prepared squash filling. Make sure to fill to the top, pressing down without puncturing the squash. In a large stockpot or rondeau with about a six-quart capacity, heat the sunflower oil on medium-high. When the oil is hot, add the stuffed squash. Fry the squash for about 7 minutes, or until it turns light brown. Remove the fried squash and place on a plate with a paper towel to absorb excess oil. Set aside.

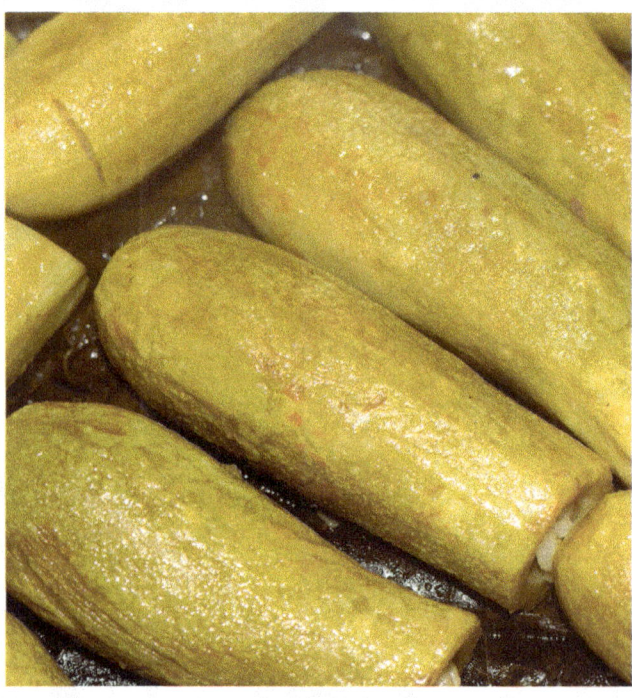

4. **Boiling the squash:** In a large stockpot or rondeau with about a five-quart capacity, bring 4 cups of the water to a boil, reduce heat to medium-low and add the fried squash. Continue to boil for 10 minutes. Remove the squash and place on a plate with paper towels to absorb moisture.

5. **Preparing the lamb chops:** Rub the lamb chops with the garlic, ½ teaspoon of the table salt, and the remaining ½ teaspoon of black pepper, ½ teaspoon of cinnamon powder, and ½ teaspoon of allspice. Place the lamb chops in a frying pan with 2½ tablespoons of the olive oil. Do not preheat the olive oil. Cook on medium heat for about 3 minutes on each side. Remove from the heat and set aside.

6. **Roasting the pine nuts:** Place the remaining ½ cup of pine nuts in a small saucepan. Add the butter and remaining 1 tablespoon of olive oil. Heat on low-medium for several minutes until the pine nuts turn light brown. Place the pine nuts on a plate, making sure to drain and discard the olive oil and butter. Set aside.

7. **Preparing the yoghurt sauce:** In a small bowl, dissolve the cornstarch with the remaining ½ cup of water, making sure that the water is cool. Add the remaining ½ teaspoon of table salt to the bowl, stir well, and set aside. Place the yoghurt in a large pan on medium heat. Using a hand whisk, stir the yoghurt in the same direction continuously. Pour the bowl of dissolved cornstarch mixture into the pan with the yoghurt. Continue to stir with the hand whisk. When the yoghurt begins to bubble, add the stuffed squash and the lamb chops. Reduce heat to low and cook for 30 to 45 minutes. At about the 35-minute mark, or 10 minutes before turning off the heat, add the roasted pine nuts. Cover the sauce and turn the heat off. Keep the sauce covered for at least 15 minutes before serving.

May be served as is or with vermicelli rice.

Cook's secret: Fry and then boil the cousa squash before adding to the yoghurt sauce.

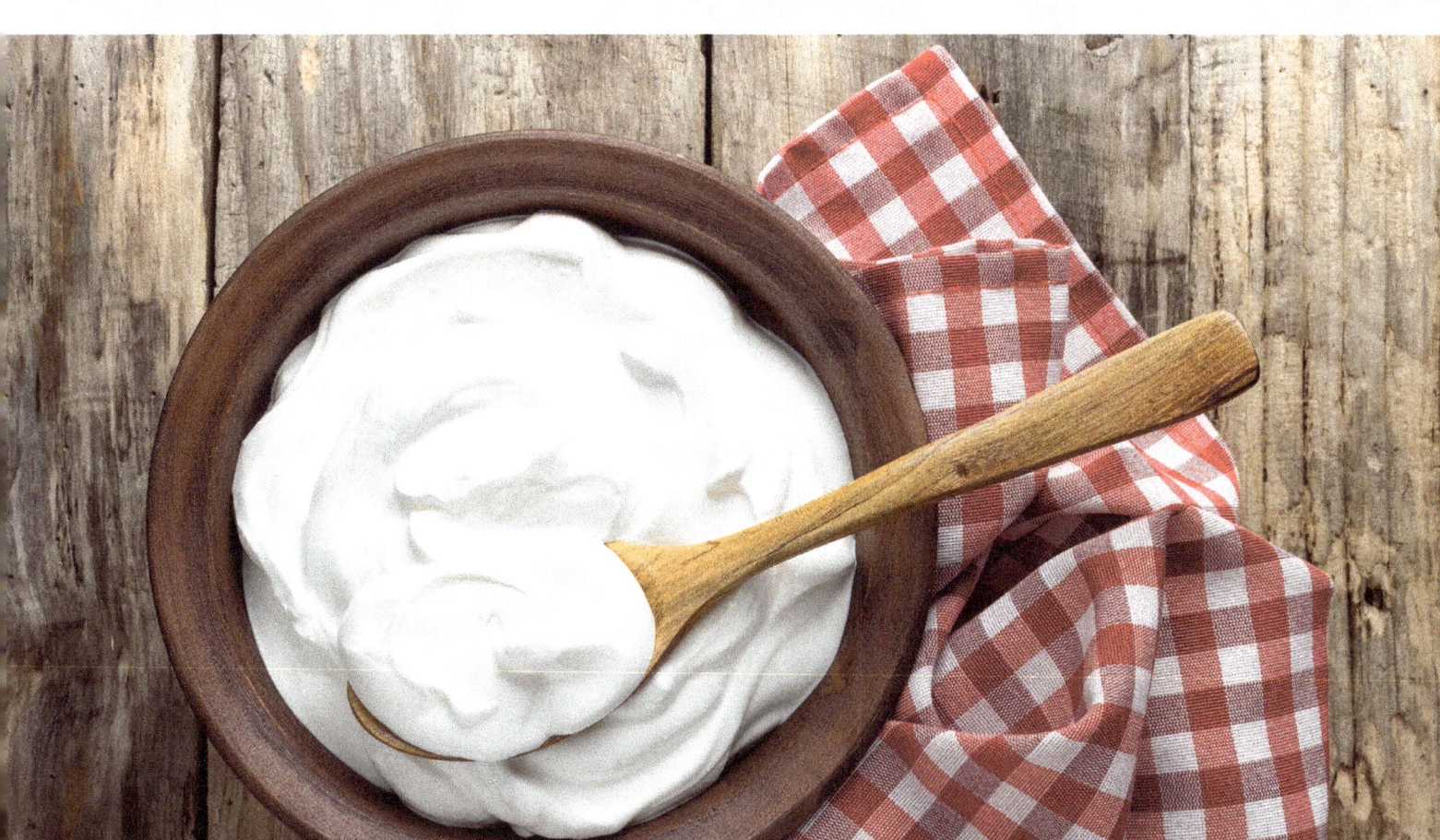

ARTICHOKE BOTTOMS STUFFED WITH MEAT

(ARDISHOWKI BI LAHM)

Serves 4–6
Total time (preparation & cooking):
1 hour, 50 minutes

---

nutritional information per serving (13.8 oz.) | **Cal** 558 **Fat** 37.5g (sat 10.7g) **Chol** 131mg **Carbs** 12g **Sugars** 1g **Protein** 44g **Fiber** 4g **Sodium** 407mg **Vit. A** (8% DV) **Vit. C** (11% DV) **Calcium** (9% DV) **Iron** (29% DV)

INGREDIENTS

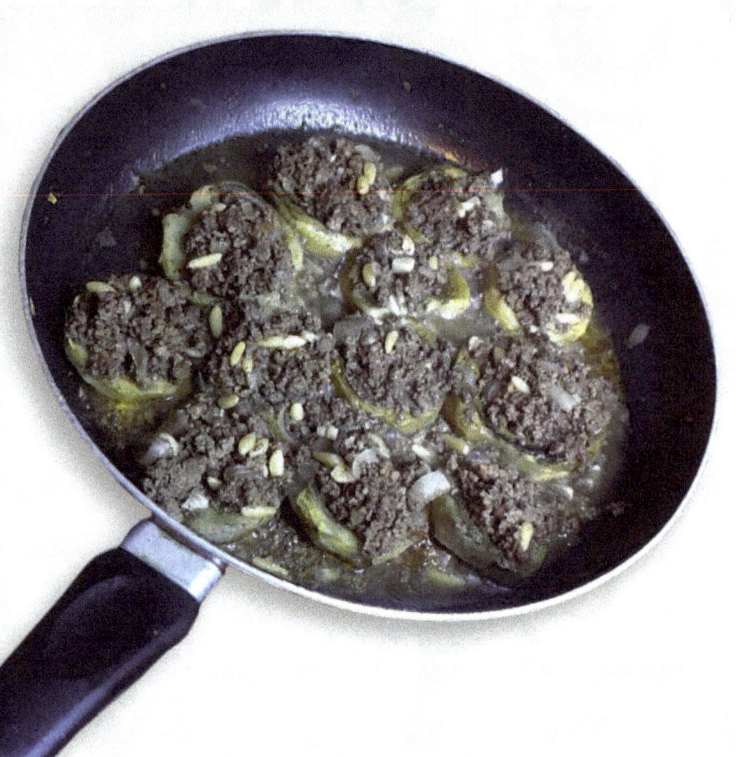

- 3 tablespoons vegetable oil (sunflower oil preferred)
- ½ stick unsalted butter (2 ounces)
- 1 (14-ounce) package frozen artichoke bottoms, thawed
- 3 tablespoons extra-virgin olive oil
- 2 pounds flank steak cut into small cubes (may substitute with sirloin steak)
- 1 medium onion, chopped
- 3 large garlic cloves, diced
- ½ teaspoon sea salt
- ¼ cup pine nuts, whole
- ½ teaspoon black pepper, coarsely ground
- 1 teaspoon cinnamon powder
- ¾ teaspoon allspice, ground
- 1 cup water
- ½ cup sour cream

INSTRUCTIONS

1. **Preparing the artichokes:** Heat up the vegetable oil and butter in a deep skillet or large saucepan. Place thawed artichoke bottoms in the skillet and cook on low-medium heat for about 15 minutes, or until they turn light golden. Set aside.

2. **Stuffing and cooking the artichokes:** In a frying pan, add the olive oil and stir in the cubed steak. Cook for about 5 minutes on low-medium heat. Add the onions, garlic cloves, sea salt, pine nuts, black pepper, cinnamon powder, and allspice. Continue to cook for 15 more minutes, stirring occasionally. Then fill each of the prepared artichoke bottoms in the skillet with the cubed steak stuffing.

   In a small bowl, mix the water and sour cream together before pouring them over the stuffed artichokes. Cover and cook in the skillet on low heat for 45 minutes. At the 30-minute mark, check to make sure that there is sufficient liquid. Add water if needed.

   May be served as is or with rice.

   Cook's secret: Use sour cream to coat the stuffed artichoke bottoms before cooking.

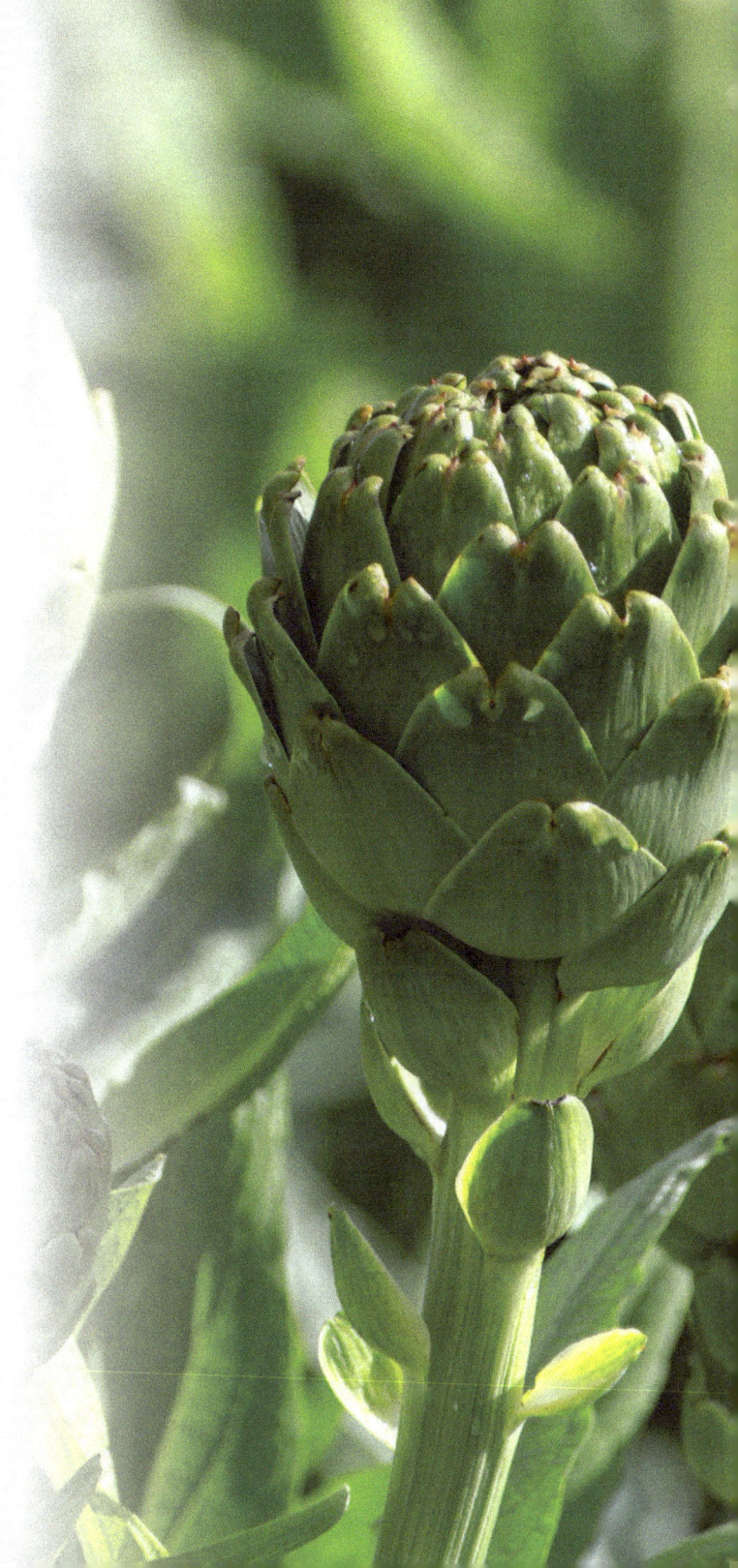

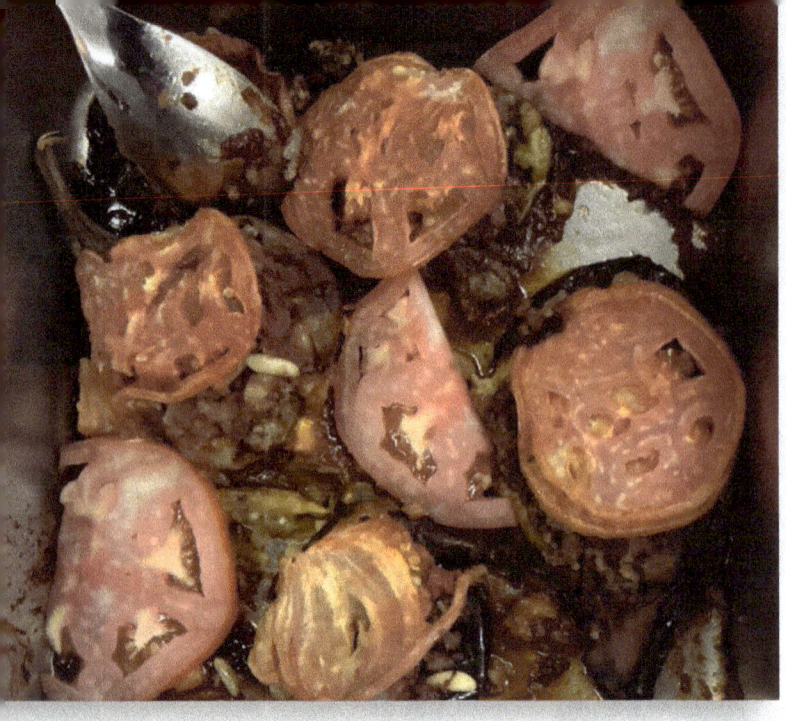

EGGPLANT STUFFED WITH MEAT

(SHEIKH EL MAHSHI)

Serves 4–6

Total time (preparation & cooking): 2 hours

---

nutritional information per serving (29.1 oz.) — **Cal** 461 **Fat** 21.5g (sat 3.8g) **Chol** 60mg **Carbs** 48g **Sugars** 27g **Protein** 27g **Fiber** 22g **Sodium** 310mg **Vit. A** (6% DV) **Vit. C** (35% DV) **Calcium** (9% DV) **Iron** (22% DV)

INGREDIENTS

- 6–7 small eggplants
- 4 tablespoons extra-virgin olive oil
- 1 large onion, diced
- 3 garlic cloves, peeled and mashed
- 1 pound ground sirloin or lamb (ground sirloin preferred)
- 1 teaspoon cinnamon powder
- ¾ teaspoon black pepper, coarsely ground
- ¾ teaspoon allspice, ground
- ½ teaspoon sea salt
- ¼ cup pine nuts, whole
- 1 cup water
- ¼ cup fresh pomegranate seeds (may substitute with 1½ tablespoons pomegranate molasses if fresh pomegranate unavailable)
- 1½ tablespoons tomato paste
- 2 medium tomatoes, cut into thin disks

INSTRUCTIONS

1. **Preparing the eggplant:** Wash the eggplant, carefully removing the stems. Partially peel the skin by leaving 3-inch-long strips. Place the eggplant in the oven in a rectangular baking pan with 1 tablespoon of the olive oil. Bake at 350°F for 15 to 25 minutes, or until the eggplant is soft enough to stuff. Cut each eggplant in half lengthwise and set aside for stuffing.

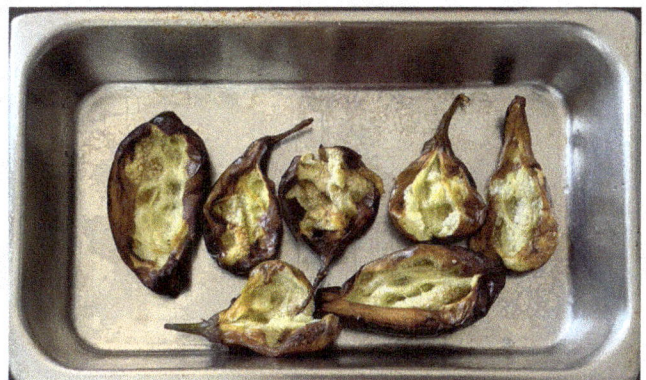

2. **Preparing the meat stuffing:** In a medium skillet, heat the remaining 3 tablespoons of olive oil. Add the onions and sauté for a few minutes on medium heat before adding the garlic. Cook for another 2 minutes and add the ground meat. Use a wooden spoon to break up the ground meat as it is cooking. Stir in the cinnamon powder, black pepper, allspice, sea salt, and pine nuts. Continue to cook for about 15 minutes, or until the meat is lightly browned. In a separate small bowl, combine the water, pomegranate seeds, and tomato paste. Mix and pour directly into the skillet. Stir and cook for 5 minutes more. Set aside.

3. **Stuffing and baking the eggplant:** Fill each eggplant with the prepared meat stuffing, leaving a small portion of the stuffing (with juices) to pour over the entire eggplant dish (for flavor and to prevent sticking). Arrange the tomatoes on top of the eggplants. Bake at 350°F for 35 to 40 minutes, or until the eggplant is cooked.

May be served as is or with rice.

Cook's secret: Use fresh pomegranate seeds in the stuffing.

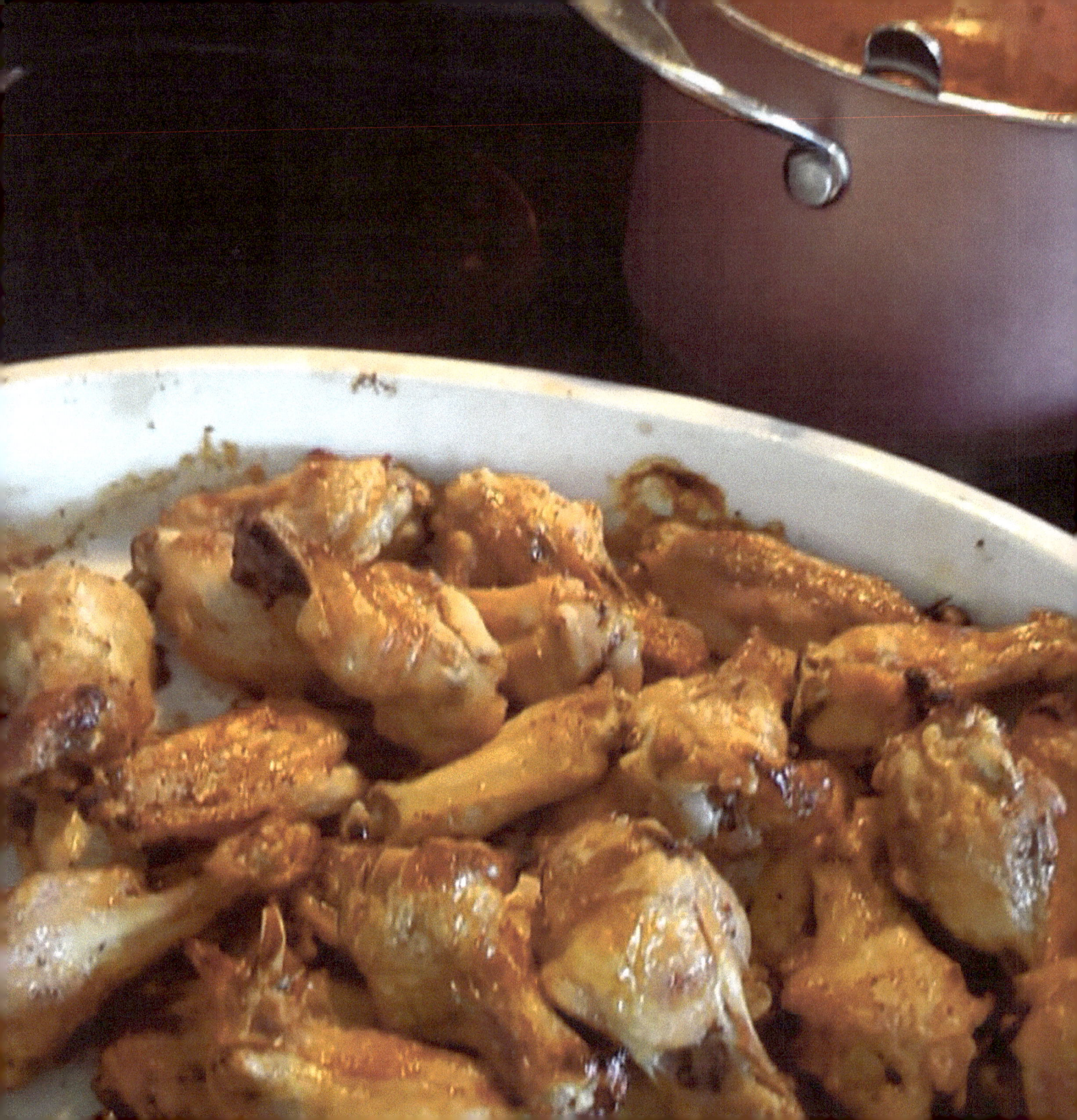

Meat, Poultry & Fish

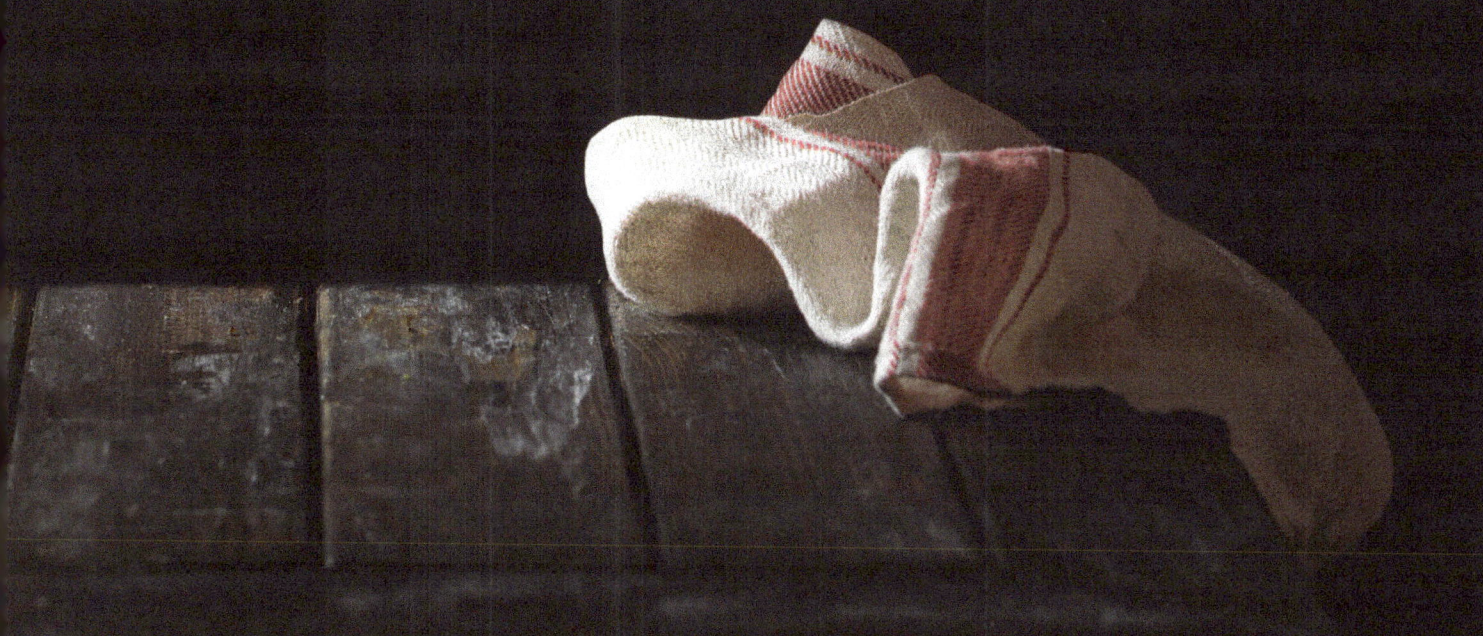

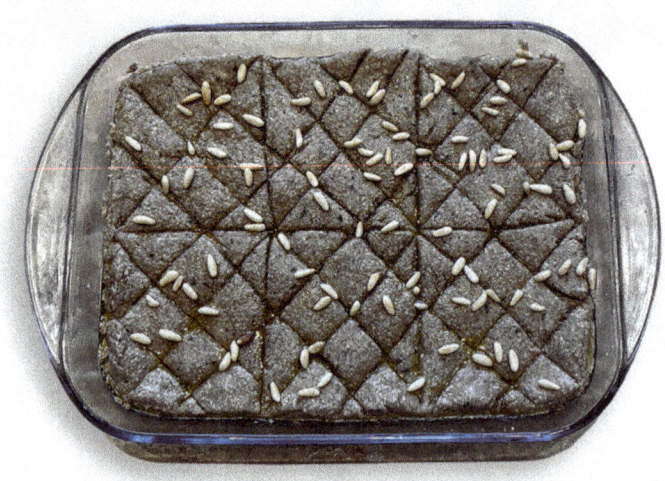

BAKED KIBBEH

Serves 4–6
Total time (preparation & cooking):
2 hours, 30 minutes

---

nutritional information per serving (15.4 oz.)

Cal 940 **Fat** 71g (sat 17.1g) **Chol** 167mg **Carbs** 21g **Sugars** 4g **Protein** 60g **Fiber** 5g **Sodium** 1030mg **Vit. A** (5% DV) **Vit. C** (11% DV) **Calcium** (6% DV) **Iron** (29% DV)

INGREDIENTS

Kibbeh stuffing

- 9 tablespoons extra-virgin olive oil
- 2 medium onions, diced
- 1½ pounds ground lamb or beef (lamb preferred)
- 1 teaspoon table salt
- 1 teaspoon cinnamon powder
- 1 teaspoon allspice, ground
- 1 teaspoon black pepper, coarsely ground
- 1 cup pine nuts, whole
- ¼ cup walnuts, whole
- 1 tablespoon lemon juice (freshly squeezed or bottled)

Kibbeh dough

- 1¾ cups bulgur
- 2 pounds finely ground lamb or sirloin (lamb preferred)
- 1 large onion, finely chopped
- 1¼ teaspoons table salt
- 1½ teaspoons cinnamon powder
- 1¼ teaspoons allspice, ground
- ½ teaspoon nutmeg, ground
- ¾ cup dried basil (may substitute with fresh basil)

INSTRUCTIONS

1. **Preparing the kibbeh stuffing:** In a medium skillet, add 2 tablespoons of the olive oil and sauté the onions over medium heat for 5 minutes. Stir in the ground meat, using a wooden spoon to break up the meat as it is cooking. Add the table salt, cinnamon powder, allspice, black pepper, ½ cup of the pine nuts, and walnuts. Cook together for about 15 minutes. Add the lemon juice. Cook for another 5 minutes and set aside.

2. **Preparing the kibbeh dough:** Wash the bulgur, and let it soak for 35 to 40 minutes in a bowl of cold water. Drain and let dry. In a medium-size bowl, combine the bulgur, ground meat, chopped onion, table salt, cinnamon powder, allspice, nutmeg, and dried basil. Knead well by hand or with a food processor until a pasty, smooth dough is formed. Divide the dough into two equal portions and set aside.

3. **Baking the kibbeh:** Preheat the oven to 365°F. Coat a rectangular baking pan or dish (13 by 9 inches) with 3 tablespoons of the olive oil. Spread the first portion of kibbeh dough to cover the entire pan. The dough on the base layer should be about ¾ inches thick. Dip hands in cold water to prevent the kibbeh dough from sticking while spreading. Add the prepared kibbeh stuffing so that it evenly covers the dough on the base of the pan.

Take the second portion of kibbeh dough and spread it on top of the stuffing, wetting hands again in cold water if the dough gets sticky. The top layer of dough should also be roughly ¾ inches thick. Use wet hands to press down on the top layer to smooth and even out. Starting from the top left corner, cut the kibbeh along a diagonal to the bottom right corner. Continue to cut in diagonal lines in the same direction, leaving at least 2 inches of space between the diagonal lines. Make sure to cut through the dough to the bottom of the baking pan.

Next, starting from the top right corner, cut the kibbeh along a diagonal line to the bottom left corner. Continue to cut along diagonal lines in the same direction, leaving at least 2 inches of space between the lines. The diagonal lines should form a rhombus-shaped design.

Pour the remaining 4 tablespoons of olive oil over the kibbeh, spreading evenly over the entire dough. Sprinkle the remaining ½ cup of pine nuts on top. Bake at 365°F for 40 to 45 minutes. Serve warm.

Best served as is.

Cook's secret: Use onions in both the kibbeh dough and the stuffing.

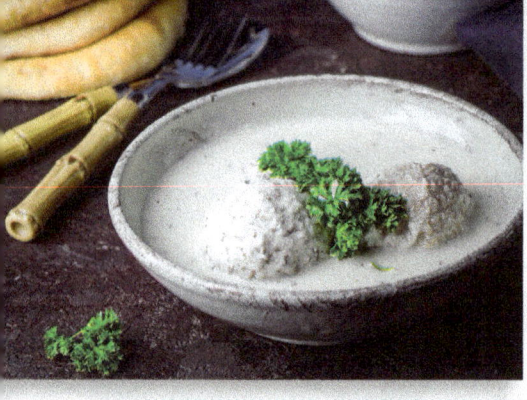

KIBBEH WITH YOGHURT SAUCE
(KIBBEH BI LABAN)

Serves 4–6
Total time (preparation & cooking): 2 hours, 40 minutes

nutritional information per serving (13.8 oz.)

Cal 657 **Fat** 48.8g (sat 13.9g) **Chol** 111mg **Carbs** 21g **Sugars** 9g **Protein** 37g **Fiber** 3g **Sodium** 952mg **Vit. A** (8% DV) **Vit. C** (9% DV) **Calcium** (22% DV) **Iron** (16% DV)

INGREDIENTS

Kibbeh stuffing
- ¼ cup extra-virgin olive oil
- 2 medium onions, finely chopped
- 1 pound ground lamb or beef (lamb preferred)
- 1 teaspoon table salt
- 1 teaspoon cinnamon powder
- 1 teaspoon allspice, ground
- ½ teaspoon nutmeg, ground
- 1 teaspoon black pepper, coarsely ground
- ¼ cup walnuts, whole
- ½ cup pine nuts, whole
- 1 teaspoon lemon juice (freshly squeezed or bottled)

Kibbeh dough
- 1 cup bulgur
- 1½ pounds finely ground lamb (may substitute with equal parts of ground lamb and ground sirloin)
- 1 medium onion, finely chopped
- 1¼ teaspoons table salt
- 1½ teaspoons cinnamon powder
- 1¼ teaspoons allspice, ground
- ½ teaspoon nutmeg, ground
- ¾ cup dried basil
- 4 tablespoons extra-virgin olive oil

Garlic sauce
- 2 tablespoons sunflower oil
- 2 tablespoons unsalted butter
- 5 garlic cloves, peeled and mashed

Yoghurt sauce
- 2½ pounds plain whole milk yoghurt
- ½ teaspoon table salt
- 3 tablespoons cornstarch
- 4 tablespoons water
- 2 teaspoons dried mint

INSTRUCTIONS

1. **Preparing the kibbeh stuffing:** In a medium skillet, add the olive oil and sauté the onions for 5 minutes on medium heat. Add the ground meat and cook for 5 minutes. Use a wooden spoon to break up the ground meat as it is cooking. Add the table salt, cinnamon powder, allspice, nutmeg, black pepper, walnuts, pine nuts, and lemon juice. Cook for another 15 to 20 minutes. Remove from the heat and set aside.

2. **Preparing the kibbeh dough for filling and baking:** Wash the bulgur, and let it soak in a bowl of cold water for 35 to 40 minutes. Drain and let dry. In a medium-size bowl, combine the bulgur, ground meat, onion, table salt, cinnamon powder, allspice, nutmeg, and dried basil. Knead well by hand or with a food processor for several minutes. Dip hands in cold water to prevent the kibbeh dough from sticking. Take enough of the dough to shape it into a large eggshell. Using your index finger, puncture one end of the kibbeh shell, creating enough space for the stuffing. The shell should be about ½ inch thick. Fill the punctured kibbeh shell with the meat stuffing (about 1 tablespoon). Close the top of the shell so that it takes the shape of either a mini football or a large teardrop. Place the shell in a baking pan greased with olive oil. Repeat the process of shaping and filling the kibbeh shells until all the dough is used. Bake the shells at 365ºF for 15 minutes. Remove from the oven and set aside. Uncooked kibbeh shells can be frozen for future use. (Kibbeh shells may also be deep-fried in vegetable oil on high heat for 10 minutes, or until light golden.)

3. **Preparing the garlic sauce:** In a separate saucepan, heat the sunflower oil and butter on low. Add the garlic, cooking on low heat until it turns light or medium brown. Remove from the heat and set aside.

4. **Preparing the yoghurt sauce for cooking the kibbeh shells:** Place the yoghurt in a medium bowl. Stir the yoghurt vigorously for about 5 minutes, or until it is smooth in texture. Add the table salt and stir to mix. In a separate small bowl, dissolve the cornstarch with the water, making sure that the water is cool. Add the dissolved cornstarch to the bowl containing the yoghurt and salt, stirring for another few minutes. Use a hand whisk to ensure that the cornstarch is fully dissolved and the yoghurt is smooth and creamy.

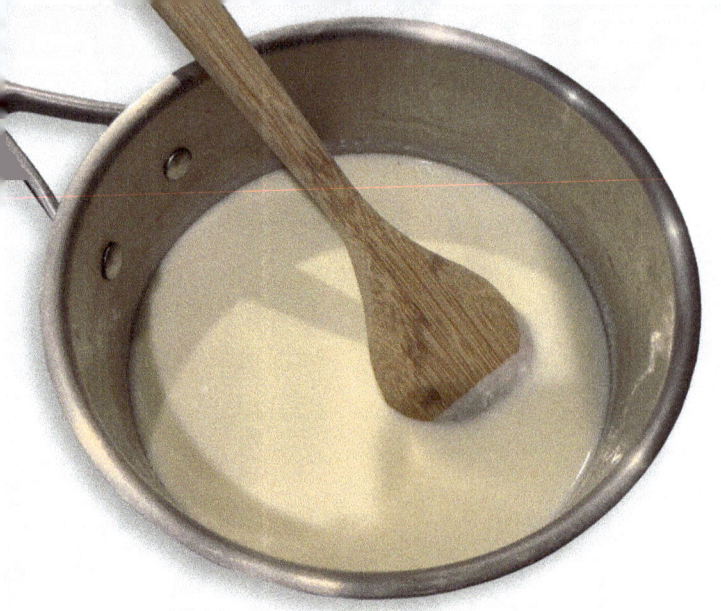

heat. Stir in the cooked garlic sauce and dried mint. Cook for an additional 5 to 7 minutes uncovered. Remove from the heat. Cover the stockpot and allow to sit for 15 minutes before serving.

Best served as is.

Cook's secret: Add the dissolved cornstarch to the yoghurt, and only add the kibbeh shells after the yoghurt sauce begins to bubble.

Pour the contents into a stockpot or rondeau with about a five-quart capacity. Cook on medium heat, stirring constantly. As soon as the yoghurt begins to boil, add the baked kibbeh shells to the yoghurt sauce. Cook the shells uncovered for 15 minutes on low

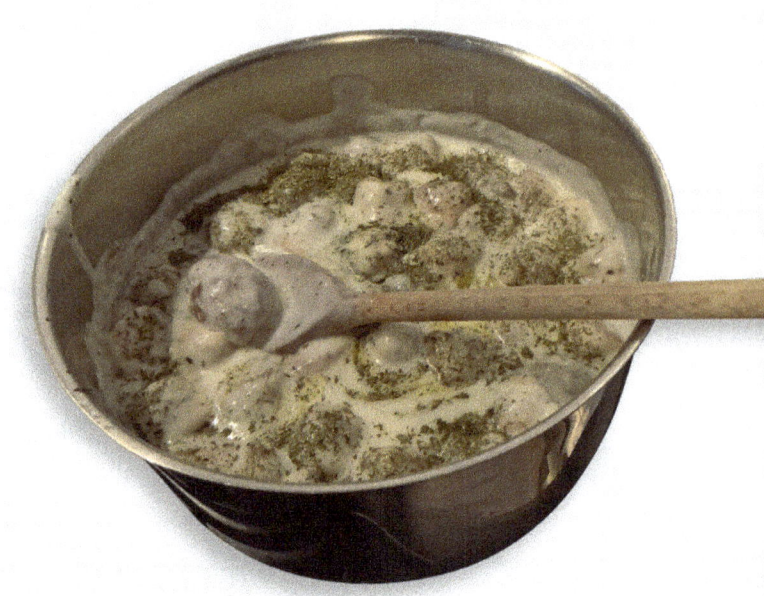

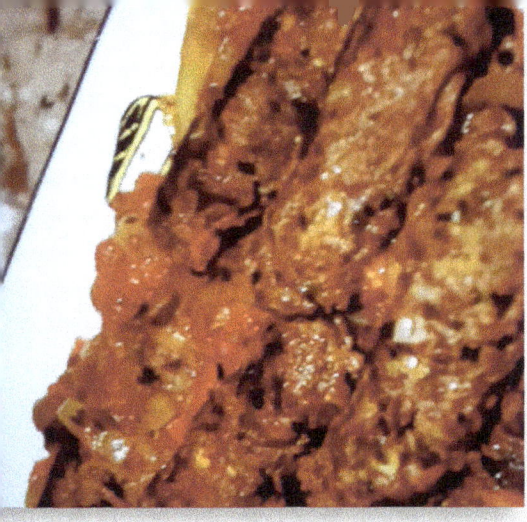

GARLIC AND PEPPER KAFTA

Serves 4–5
Total time (preparation & cooking): 1 hour, 40 minutes

nutritional information per serving (7.1 oz.) — **Cal** 531 **Fat** 45.3g (sat 17.2g) **Chol** 95mg **Carbs** 6g **Sugars** 3g **Protein** 24g **Fiber** 1g **Sodium** 659mg **Vit. A** (12% DV) **Vit. C** (175% DV) **Calcium** (3% DV) **Iron** (18% DV)

INGREDIENTS

- 1½ pounds ground or very finely chopped boneless short rib
- 3 fresh hot red peppers, finely chopped with seeds removed
- 3 fresh hot green peppers, finely chopped with seeds removed
- 5 garlic cloves, peeled and mashed
- 1 teaspoon black pepper, coarsely ground
- 1 teaspoons sea salt
- 2 tablespoons extra-virgin olive oil

INSTRUCTIONS

1. **Preparing and baking the *kafta*:** Place the ground short rib meat in a large bowl. Add the hot red peppers and green peppers. Mix by hand to combine, squeezing the juices from the peppers while kneading the meat. Add the garlic, black pepper, and sea salt. Continue to mix by hand. Once the kafta is well kneaded, let it sit for 30 minutes to 1 hour in the fridge. Remove from the fridge and shape kafta into 6-inch-long links (like sausage links). Place kafta links in a baking dish or pan. Drizzle the olive oil over the kafta and bake in a preheated oven at 350ºF for 30 minutes.

May also be served grilled or fried in a skillet over medium heat.

Cook's secret: Squeeze juices from the chopped hot peppers while kneading the rib meat.

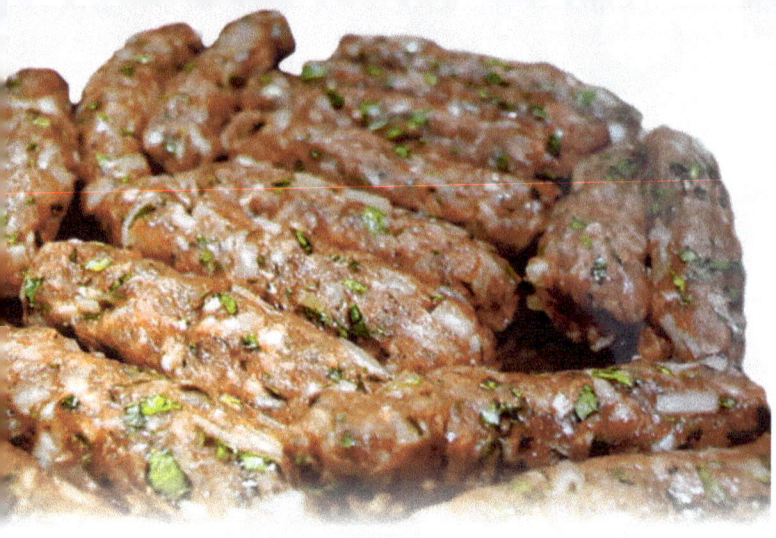

CLASSIC KAFTA

Serves 4–5

Total time (preparation & cooking): 1 hour

---

nutritional information per serving (8.4 oz.) **Cal** 344 **Fat** 22.6g (sat 7.4g) **Chol** 86mg **Carbs** 7g **Sugars** 3g **Protein** 29g **Fiber** 2g **Sodium** 560mg **Vit. A** (47% DV) **Vit. C** (65% DV) **Calcium** (6% DV) **Iron** (19% DV)

INGREDIENTS

- 1 bunch Italian flat parsley, finely chopped
- 1 bunch fresh mint, finely chopped
- ¾ pound ground lamb
- ¾ pound ground beef
- 1 medium onion, very finely chopped
- 1 teaspoon black pepper, coarsely ground
- 1 teaspoon sea salt
- 2 tablespoons extra-virgin olive oil

Side garnish

- 1 bunch Italian flat parsley, finely chopped
- 1 bunch fresh mint, finely chopped
- 1 tomato, diced
- 1 medium onion, sliced lengthwise into strips
- ½ teaspoon sumac
- 1 fresh hot red pepper with seeds removed (optional)
- ½ teaspoon black pepper, coarsely ground
- 1 loaf pita bread (optional)
- 2 tablespoons extra-virgin olive oil (optional)

INSTRUCTIONS

1. **Preparing and baking the *kafta*:** Place the chopped parsley (without stems) and chopped mint in a medium bowl. Fill the bowl with water. Drain using a fine mesh sieve. Repeat this process several times to remove all the dirt. In a separate large bowl, use hands to combine the well-drained parsley and mint with the ground lamb and ground beef. Add the chopped onion, black pepper, and sea salt. Use the palm of the hand to mix and knead the meat for about 4 minutes, or until it is soft and elastic. Shape the kafta into 6-inch-long links (like sausage links) and place in a large baking dish or pan. Drizzle the olive oil over the kafta and bake in a preheated oven at 350°F for 30 minutes, or until the meat is cooked. Kafta may also be grilled or fried in a skillet over medium heat.

2. **Preparing the side garnish:** Place the chopped parsley (without stems) and mint in a medium bowl. Fill the bowl with water. Drain using a fine mesh sieve. Repeat this process several times to remove all the dirt. In a separate large bowl, combine the well-drained parsley and mint with the tomato, diced onion, sumac, hot red pepper (if desired), and black pepper.

   If serving without pita bread, add olive oil to the bowl, stir, and set aside. If serving with pita bread, form a pocket by partially opening or peeling apart the bread halfway, and drizzle the olive oil on one side of the interior pocket. Spread the prepared garnish over the oil. Toast closed face in a preheated oven at 350°F for 5 to 8 minutes, or until the bread is lightly browned.

   May be served with the garnish on the side or with the garnish toasted in the pita bread.

   Cook's secret: Knead the ground lamb and beef mixture by hand until all ingredients are well incorporated and the meat texture is smooth.

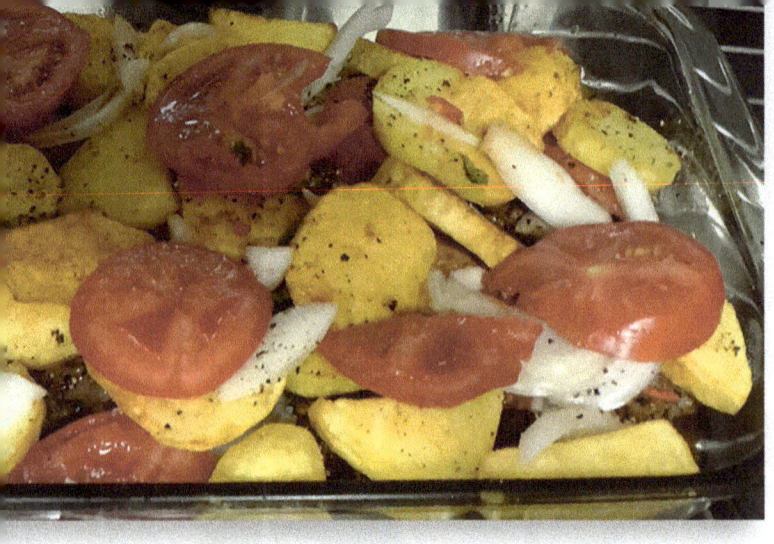

ALL-SPICES KAFTA

Serves 4–6
Total time (preparation & cooking):
1 hour, 40 minutes

nutritional information per serving (8.7 oz.)	**Cal** 408 **Fat** 25.3g (sat 7.8g) **Chol** 86mg **Carbs** 17g **Sugars** 2g **Protein** 30g **Fiber** 3g **Sodium** 550mg **Vit. A** (8% DV) **Vit. C** (29% DV) **Calcium** (3% DV) **Iron** (14% DV)

INGREDIENTS

1	large potato, peeled	½	teaspoon cinnamon powder
1½	pounds ground lamb	½	teaspoon cumin, ground
1	white onion, very finely chopped	½	teaspoon black pepper, coarsely ground
1	bunch fresh mint, finely chopped	1	teaspoon sea salt
3	garlic cloves, peeled and mashed	3	tablespoons extra-virgin olive oil
½	teaspoon cardamom, ground	1	large tomato, sliced into thin disks
1	teaspoon paprika	1	medium onion, sliced lengthwise
½	teaspoon red pepper		

INSTRUCTIONS

1. **Preparing the potato:** Boil water in a medium saucepan. Add the potato and boil for 25 minutes. Drain water and allow potato to cool. Slice the potato into disks (about ¾ inch thick) and set aside.

2. **Preparing and baking the *kafta*:** In a large bowl, combine the ground lamb with the onion, mint, garlic, cardamom, paprika, red pepper, cinnamon powder, cumin, black pepper, sea salt, and 1 tablespoon of the olive oil. Knead with hands for several minutes to combine. Place the kafta in the fridge for 1 hour. Remove from the fridge and shape into round hamburger-like patties. Space the kafta patties about an inch apart in a baking dish or pan. Cover the patties with the prepared potato disks. Add the sliced tomato and onion, arranging them evenly over the patties before drizzling the remaining 2 tablespoons of olive oil on top. Bake in a preheated oven at 350°F for about 35 minutes.

May also be served grilled or fried in a skillet over medium heat.

Cook's secret: Blend the cardamom, cinnamon, and cumin and use fresh mint.

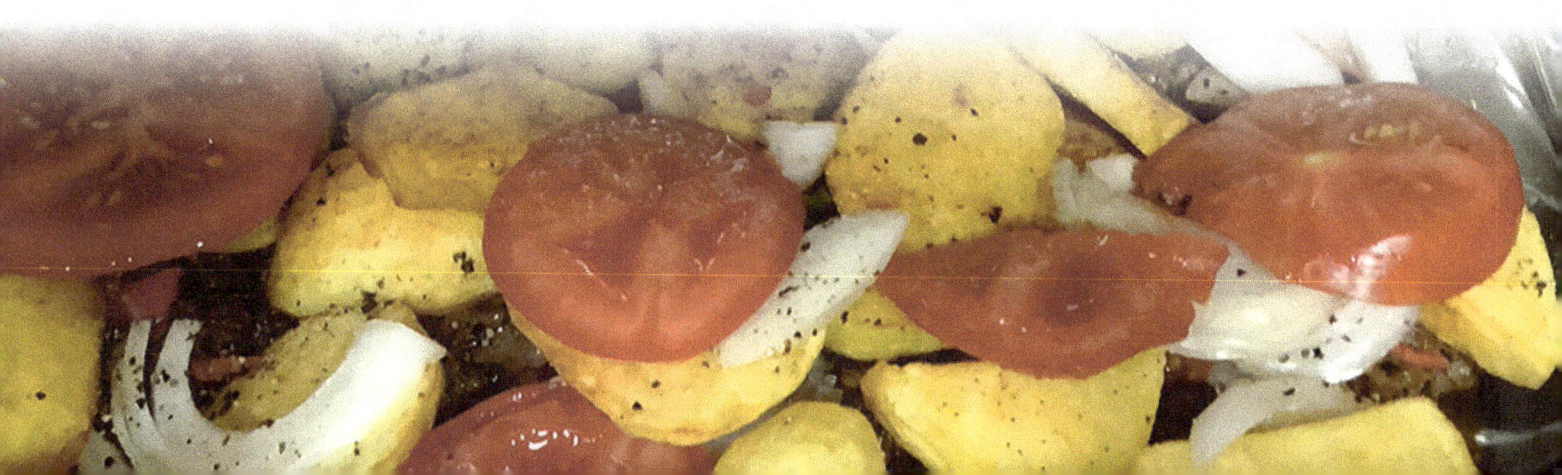

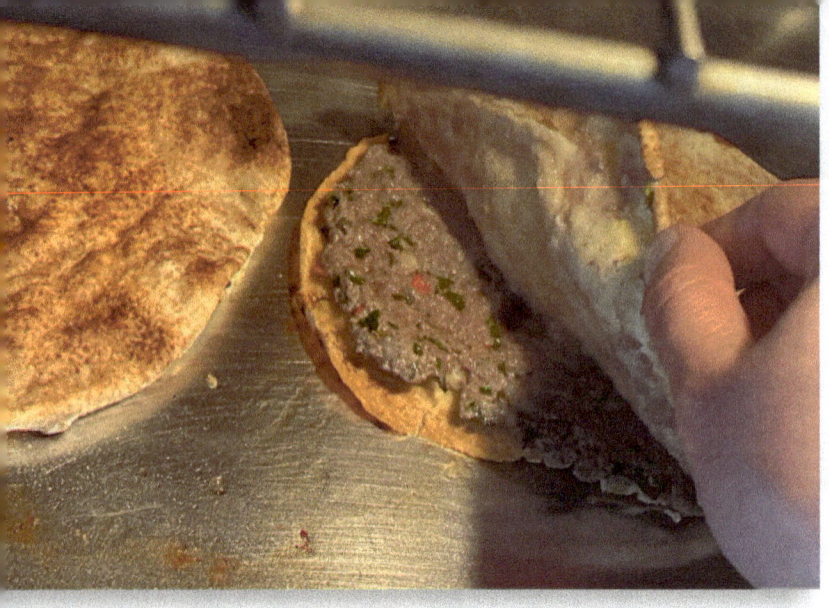

SWEET AND SPICY KAFTA

Serves 4–6
Total time (preparation & cooking):
2 hours, 45 minutes

---

nutritional information per serving (10.2 oz.) — **Cal** 461 **Fat** 23.7g (sat 7g) **Chol** 86mg **Carbs** 32g **Sugars** 10g **Protein** 32g **Fiber** 4g **Sodium** 488mg **Vit. A** (28% DV) **Vit. C** (83% DV) **Calcium** (7% DV) **Iron** (21% DV)

INGREDIENTS

- 1 bunch Italian flat parsley, finely chopped
- 1 bunch fresh mint, finely chopped
- 1½ pounds ground lamb
- 1 large white onion, finely chopped
- 2 fresh hot red peppers, finely chopped with seeds removed
- 1 teaspoon cumin, ground
- 1 teaspoon chili powder
- 1 teaspoon coriander, ground
- 2 tablespoons pomegranate molasses
- 1 teaspoon table salt
- 2 tablespoons extra-virgin olive oil
- 4–6 loaves of pita bread (optional)

INSTRUCTIONS

1. **Preparing and baking the *kafta*:** Place the chopped parsley (without stems) and chopped mint in a medium bowl. Fill the bowl with water. Drain using a fine mesh sieve. Repeat this process several times to remove all the dirt. In a separate large bowl, combine the well-drained parsley and mint with the ground lamb, onion, hot red peppers, cumin, chili powder, coriander, pomegranate molasses, and table salt. Knead with hands until all the ingredients are well combined. Place the kafta in the fridge for 2 hours before baking. To bake without bread, shape the kafta into 6-inch-long links (like sausage links) and place in a baking dish or pan. Preheat the oven to 350°F. Drizzle the olive oil over the kafta and bake for about 35 minutes.

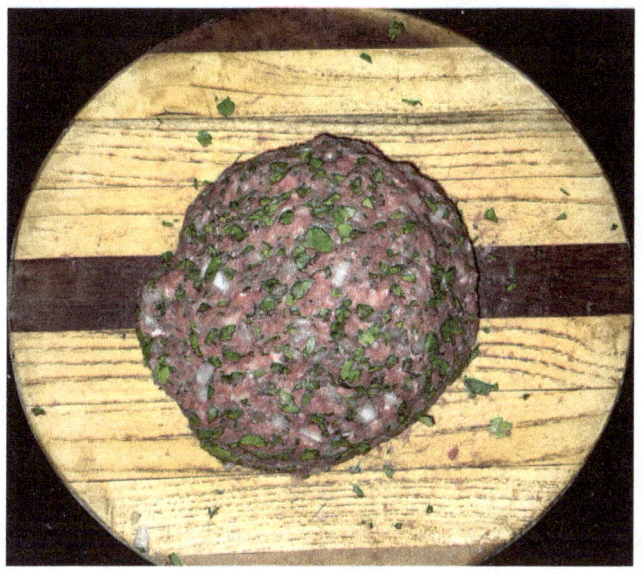

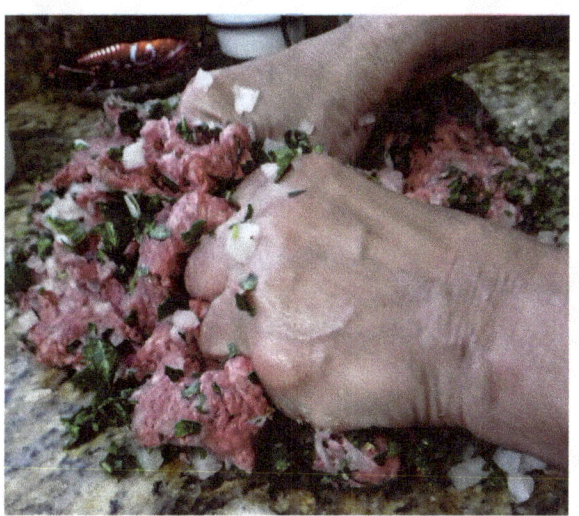

If serving with pita bread, bake the kafta inside the pita pocket by partially opening or peeling apart the bread halfway and spreading a thin layer of kafta onto one side of the interior pocket. Toast closed face in a preheated oven at 350ºF for 13 to 15 minutes.

May also be served grilled or fried in a skillet over medium heat.

Cook's secret: Blend the pomegranate molasses with the hot spices.

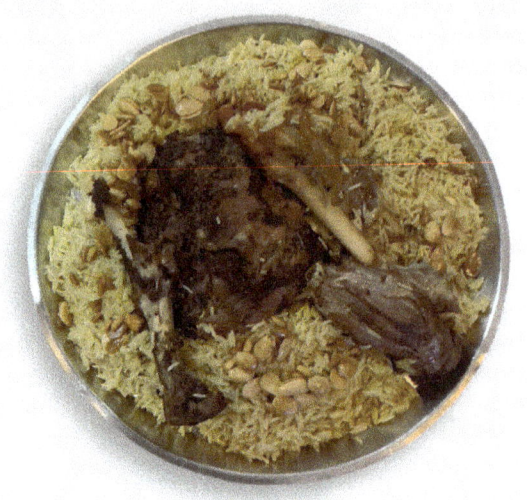

LEBANESE LAMB WITH RICE

Serves 4–6
Total time (preparation & cooking):
4 hours, 45 minutes

---

nutritional information per serving (15.8 oz.) — **Cal** 721 **Fat** 43.9g (sat 15.9g) **Chol** 91mg **Carbs** 58g **Sugars** 1g **Protein** 21g **Fiber** 4g **Sodium** 1145mg **Vit. A** (11% DV) **Vit. C** (7% DV) **Calcium** (8% DV) **Iron** (22% DV)

INGREDIENTS

- 1 leg of lamb
- 2 cups distilled white vinegar
- 1 stick unsalted butter (4 ounces, or ¼ pound), melted
- 3 tablespoons fresh lemon zest
- 1½ teaspoons cinnamon powder
- 1 teaspoon black pepper, coarsely ground
- 1 teaspoon allspice, ground
- ½ teaspoon nutmeg, ground
- 1 teaspoon garlic powder
- 2 tablespoons dried onion powder
- 2 teaspoons table salt
- ¼ cup red wine
- 6 cardamom, whole
- 1 cinnamon stick
- 3½ cups water

Rice and beef

- 2 cups white basmati rice (may substitute with medium-grain Egyptian white rice)
- 2 tablespoons extra-virgin olive oil
- 1½ cups ground beef
- ½ teaspoon table salt
- ½ teaspoon black pepper, coarsely ground
- ½ teaspoon cinnamon powder
- 1 teaspoon allspice, ground
- ¼ cup pine nuts, whole

Garnish

- 2 tablespoons unsalted butter
- 1 tablespoon extra-virgin olive oil
- ¾ cup raw almonds, peeled and whole
- ½ cup pine nuts, whole

INSTRUCTIONS

1. **Preparing and baking the lamb:** Wash the leg of lamb with the distilled white vinegar. Pat the lamb dry with a paper towel and place in a deep baking pan. Rub the melted butter, lemon zest, cinnamon powder, black pepper, allspice, nutmeg, garlic powder, dried onion powder, and table salt over the lamb, evenly coating all sides. Add the red wine, cardamom, and cinnamon stick. Pour the water into the pan and cover with aluminum foil, sealing tightly. Preheat the oven to 350ºF and bake for 3 hours, or until the lamb is tender. Carefully remove the foil. Save the lamb stock for the rice and beef mixture.

2. **Preparing the rice and beef mixture:** Rinse the rice, drain, and set aside. In a large saucepan, add the olive oil and ground beef. Cook on low-medium heat, using a wooden spoon to break up the beef. Gradually add the salt, black pepper, cinnamon powder, and allspice. Once the ground beef has turned light brown, add the pine nuts. Then pour in 3 ½ cups of the prepared lamb stock and bring to a boil. If there is insufficient lamb stock left, use water instead. Stir in the rinsed rice and immediately reduce heat to low. Cover and cook for 35 to 40 minutes on low heat. Remove from the heat and keep covered for 10 minutes before serving.

3. **Preparing the garnish:** In a separate frying pan, heat the butter and olive oil. Add the almonds, toasting until they begin to change color. Stir in the pine nuts and continue to fry until both the pine nuts and almonds turn golden brown.

Best served with the lamb over the rice topped with the nut garnish.

Cook's secret: Use lemon zest with the lamb, and tightly seal the lamb while it is cooking.

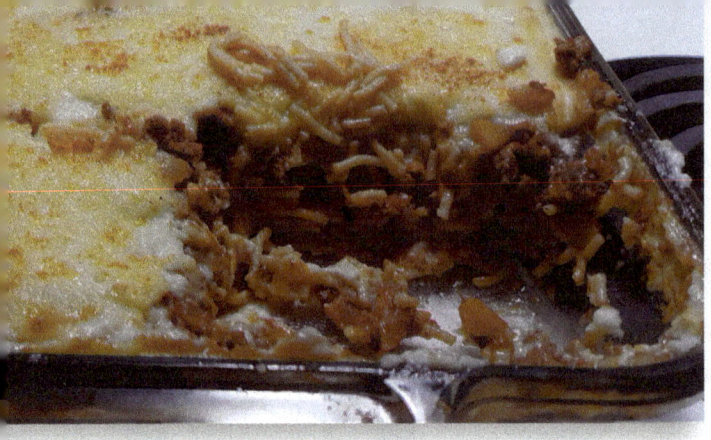

LEBANESE SPAGHETTI WITH BÉCHAMEL

(MACARONI BI HALIB)

Serves 6
Total time (preparation & cooking): 3 hours

---

nutritional information per serving (22.7 oz.) — **Cal** 685 **Fat** 35g (sat 15.4g) **Chol** 139mg **Carbs** 47g **Sugars** 15g **Protein** 48g **Fiber** 6g **Sodium** 1219mg **Vit. A** (123% DV) **Vit. C** (22% DV) **Calcium** (46% DV) **Iron** (20% DV)

INGREDIENTS

- 3 tablespoons extra-virgin olive oil
- 1 onion, diced
- 4 garlic cloves, peeled and mashed
- 3 medium carrots, finely chopped
- 3 celery stalks, finely chopped
- 2 pounds ground lamb or beef (lamb preferred)
- 1½ teaspoons table salt
- 1 teaspoon dried oregano
- 1 teaspoon thyme
- 1 teaspoon black pepper, coarsely ground
- 1 teaspoon dried basil (may substitute with ½ cup freshly chopped basil)
- ½ cup red wine
- 2 tablespoons tomato paste
- 1 can plum tomatoes (may substitute with 5 fresh plum tomatoes, chopped)
- ½ cup tomato juice, freshly squeezed
- 1 cup water
- 1 (16-ounce) package spaghetti

Béchamel sauce

- 5 cups whole milk (may substitute with reduced fat milk)
- 4½ tablespoons cornstarch
- 1 toothpick
- 1 bay leaf
- 1 halved onion, un-chopped
- 1 cup grated Parmesan cheese
- 3 tablespoons salted butter
- 4 cloves, whole
- ½ teaspoon black pepper, coarsely ground
- ¼ teaspoon nutmeg, ground

INSTRUCTIONS

1. **Preparing the ground meat sauce:** In a large stockpot or rondeau with a six-quart capacity, heat the olive oil on low-medium. Add the onions and sauté for 3 minutes. Add the garlic, carrots, and celery, cooking for 4 minutes more. Add the ground meat, 1 teaspoon of the table salt, oregano, thyme, black pepper, and basil. Continue cooking on low-medium heat until the meat turns light brown. Stir in the red wine and mix well. Add the tomato paste, plum tomatoes, and tomato juice. Stir in the water and reduce heat to low. Cook the sauce on low heat for 45 minutes to 1 hour. Check on the sauce every 30 minutes to ensure that there is sufficient liquid. If the sauce appears dry, add more water.

2. **Preparing the béchamel sauce:** In a bowl, combine the milk and cornstarch. Whisk together by hand until the cornstarch dissolves. Place the mixture in a saucepan on low-medium heat. Using a toothpick, attach the bay leaf to the halved onion and place it in the saucepan. Add ½ cup of the grated Parmesan cheese and butter, stirring constantly with a wooden spoon. Add the cloves, black pepper, and nutmeg. Continue stirring and cook until the sauce begins to thicken, about 20 minutes. Discard the onion with bay leaf. Remove the sauce from the heat and set aside.

3. **Preparing the spaghetti:** In a large pan, bring water to a boil. Add the spaghetti and the remaining ½ teaspoon of table salt. Boil for 7 minutes, or until the noodles are partially cooked. Drain and set aside.

4. **Putting it all together:** Preheat the oven to 350°F. In a large rectangular baking dish (13 by 9 inches), spread some of the meat sauce on the bottom to prevent sticking. Add the drained spaghetti. Pour the meat sauce on top of the noodles. Then pour the béchamel sauce on top, spreading evenly. Sprinkle the remaining ½ cup of grated Parmesan over the béchamel. Cook for 35 to 40 minutes. The béchamel top should turn golden brown when finished.

Best served as is.

Cook's secret: Prepare the béchamel sauce with whole cloves, onion, and bay leaf.

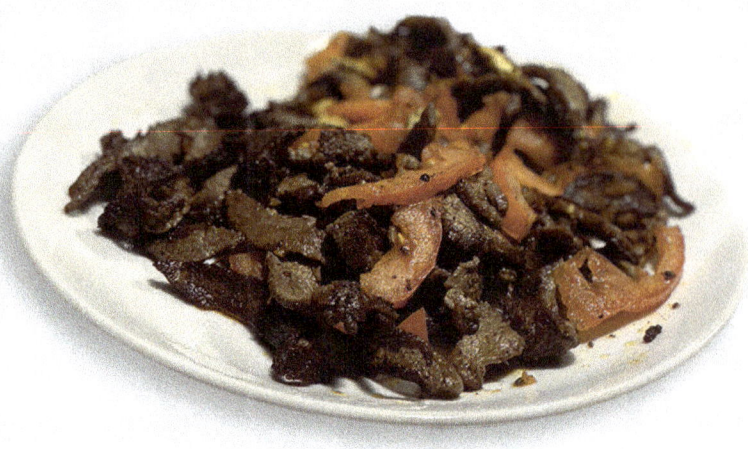

BEEF SHAWARMA

Serves 4–6
Total time (preparation & cooking):
40 minutes + 12 hours marination

> nutritional information†
> per serving (9.2 oz.)
> † includes tahini sauce
>
> **Cal** 441 **Fat** 28.1g (sat 7.9g) **Chol** 115mg **Carbs** 5g **Sugars** 1g **Protein** 41g **Fiber** 2g
> **Sodium** 694mg **Vit. A** (5% DV) **Vit. C** (14% DV) **Calcium** (10% DV) **Iron** (23% DV)

INGREDIENTS

- 2 tablespoons lemon juice (freshly squeezed or bottled)
- ¼ cup apple cider vinegar
- ¼ teaspoon cloves, ground
- 1 teaspoon table salt
- ½ teaspoon cumin, ground
- 1 teaspoon cinnamon powder
- ½ teaspoon nutmeg, ground
- ½ teaspoon black pepper, coarsely ground
- ½ teaspoon ginger powder
- ½ teaspoon cayenne
- 1 teaspoon mastic, crushed
- 2 tablespoons red wine
- 6 cardamom, whole
- 2 pounds flank beef strips, thinly sliced (may substitute with filet mignon)
- ¼ cup extra-virgin olive oil
- 2 tablespoons unsalted butter
- 2 small tomatoes, thinly sliced

Tahini sauce

- 3 tablespoons tahini (sesame paste)
- ¼ cup lemon juice (freshly squeezed or bottled)
- 2 tablespoons water
- 1 garlic clove, peeled and crushed
- ¼ teaspoon sea salt

INSTRUCTIONS

1. **Preparing the beef marinade:** In a large bowl, combine the lemon juice, apple cider vinegar, cloves, table salt, cumin, cinnamon powder, nutmeg, black pepper, ginger powder, cayenne, mastic, and red wine. Using a pestle, cup, or wooden spoon, smash the cardamom to crack open the pods and add them to the marinade. Add the beef strips to the bowl and coat thoroughly. Pour in the olive oil and mix well by hand. Cover the bowl with plastic wrap and place in the fridge for 12 to 18 hours.

2. **Cooking the beef shawarma:** Cook the marinated beef shawarma in a large frying pan on medium heat, stirring occasionally. Remove from the heat after roughly 8 minutes, or until the juices from the beef are no longer pink. Drain all the juices from the pan. Add the butter and continue to cook on medium heat. Remove from the heat when the meat turns brown, stirring in the tomatoes a few minutes beforehand so that they have a chance to cook slightly.

3. **Preparing the tahini sauce:** Combine the tahini, lemon juice, water, garlic, and sea salt. Mix thoroughly. If the sauce is too thick, add a little more water.

May be served with the tahini on the side as a dipping sauce or in a pita sandwich stuffed with pickles and french fries and topped with the tahini sauce.

Cook's secret: Remove the marination juices from the flank steak before returning to heat.

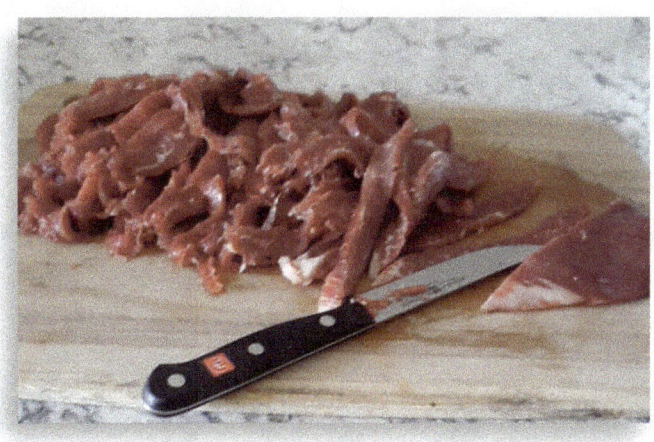

CHICKEN SHAWARMA

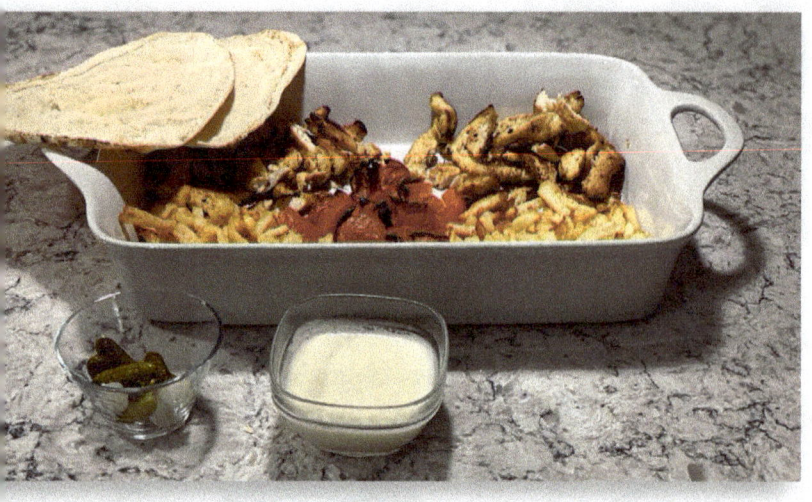

Serves 4–6
Total time (preparation & cooking):
40 minutes + 12 hours marination +
5 hours soaking

> **nutritional information**[†]
> **per serving (9.9 oz.)**
> [†] does not include garlic paste
>
> **Cal** 354 **Fat** 20.3g (sat 6.3g) **Chol** 130mg **Carbs** 5g **Sugars** 1g **Protein** 39g **Fiber** 1g **Sodium** 1088mg **Vit. A** (10% DV) **Vit. C** (17% DV) **Calcium** (7% DV) **Iron** (6% DV)

INGREDIENTS

- 1 cup buttermilk (may substitute with plain yoghurt)
- 3 tablespoons distilled white vinegar
- 2 tablespoons white wine
- ½ cup lemon juice (freshly squeezed or bottled)
- 3 tablespoons extra-virgin olive oil
- 2 teaspoons garlic powder
- 1½ teaspoons table salt
- ½ teaspoon dried oregano
- ¼ teaspoon thyme
- ½ teaspoon paprika
- ½ teaspoon ginger powder
- ½ teaspoon cayenne
- ¼ teaspoon nutmeg, ground
- ½ teaspoon mastic, ground
- ½ teaspoon dried cilantro
- 5 cardamom, whole
- 2 pounds skinless, boneless chicken breasts, thinly cut
- ½ stick unsalted butter (2 ounces)

Garlic paste

- 8 garlic cloves, cut in half
- ¼ teaspoon table salt
- 1 egg white
- ½ cup vegetable oil (sunflower oil preferred)
- 2½ tablespoons lemon juice (freshly squeezed or bottled)

INSTRUCTIONS

1. **Preparing the chicken marinade:** Rinse the chicken in cold water. Cut horizontally into long, thin pieces and set aside. To create the marinade, combine the buttermilk, distilled white vinegar, white wine, lemon juice, olive oil, garlic powder, table salt, oregano, thyme, paprika, ginger powder, cayenne, nutmeg, mastic, cilantro, and cardamom in a large mixing bowl. Using a hand whisk or food processor, mix the marinade ingredients. Add the chicken to the mixing bowl and coat the chicken with the marinade, making sure that all slices are well coated. Place the marinated chicken in the fridge overnight, or for 12 to 18 hours.

2. **Preparing the garlic paste:** Soak the garlic cloves in ice water for 5 hours. Remove the garlic and dry using a paper towel. Pulse the garlic and table salt in a food processor, preferably a Cuisinart. Add the egg white and continue to blend. Scrape down the sides of the food processor bowl using a small spatula if ingredients get stuck to the sides. Gradually add ¼ cup of the vegetable oil, leaving the food processor running. Add the lemon juice very slowly using a dropper. After dispensing a few drops of the lemon juice, stop and gradually add the remaining ¼ cup of vegetable oil. Finish adding the lemon juice with the dropper. Blend for about 5 minutes, or until a thick paste is formed. Set aside.

3. **Cooking the marinated chicken:** Place the chicken in a large frying pan on medium-high heat. Cook the chicken, stirring constantly until juices form and the chicken is no longer red or pink. Drain and discard all the juices from the chicken. Return the chicken to the frying pan, reducing heat to medium-low. Add the butter. Cook the chicken evenly for about 20 minutes, or until it turns golden brown.

May be served with the garlic paste as a spread or in a pita sandwich stuffed with pickles and french fries and topped with the garlic paste.

Cook's secret: Remove the marination juices from the chicken during the cooking process.

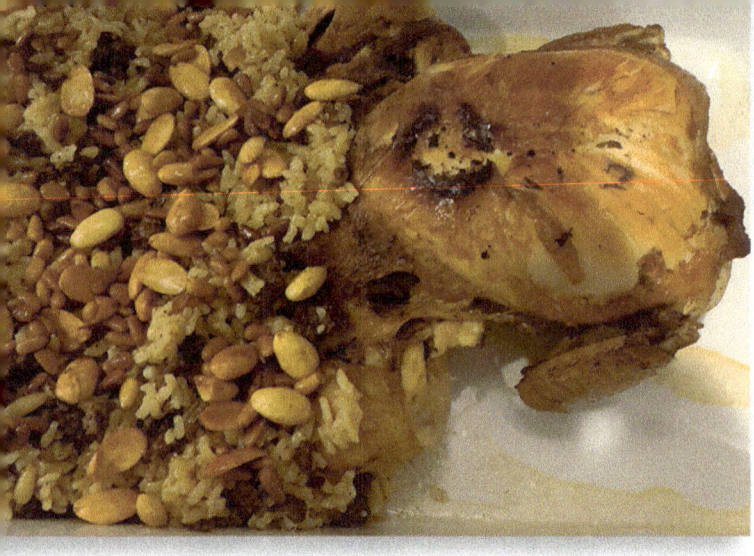

LEBANESE CHICKEN AND RICE

(RIZ BI DAJAJ)

Serves 6–8
Total time (preparation & cooking): 3 hours

> **nutritional information per serving (16.3 oz.)**
> **Cal** 717 **Fat** 36.7g (sat 8g) **Chol** 134mg **Carbs** 49g **Sugars** 3g **Protein** 48g **Fiber** 4g **Sodium** 877mg **Vit. A** (3% DV) **Vit. C** (9% DV) **Calcium** (8% DV) **Iron** (26% DV)

INGREDIENTS

- 1 whole chicken (skin-on)
- 3 tablespoons all-purpose flour
- 1 lemon, freshly squeezed
- 3 teaspoons cinnamon powder
- 2½ teaspoons allspice, ground
- 2½ teaspoons sea salt
- 2½ teaspoons black pepper, coarsely ground
- ½ teaspoon nutmeg, ground
- 4 tablespoons extra-virgin olive oil
- 3 tablespoons red wine
- 3½ cups water
- 1 cinnamon stick
- 6 cloves, whole
- 1 teaspoon turmeric
- 1 medium onion, peeled and un-chopped
- 5 garlic cloves, peeled
- 6 cardamom, whole
- 2 cups medium-grain Egyptian white rice (may substitute with white basmati rice)
- 1½ pounds ground lamb or beef (lamb preferred)
- 1 cup pine nuts, whole
- 1½ tablespoons sunflower oil (may substitute with another vegetable oil)
- 1½ tablespoons unsalted butter
- ¾ cup raw almonds, peeled and whole

INSTRUCTIONS

1. **Cleaning the chicken:** Scrub the chicken with the flour and ½ squeezed lemon. Rinse thoroughly with cold water. Let the chicken dry.

2. **Spicing the chicken:** Rub the chicken with 2 teaspoons of the cinnamon powder, 1½ teaspoons of the allspice, 1½ teaspoons of the sea salt, 1½ teaspoons of the black pepper, and the nutmeg.

3. **Preparing the chicken and chicken stock:** In a large stockpot or rondeau with about a six-quart capacity, heat 2½ tablespoons of the olive oil. Place the chicken in the pot and reduce heat to low. Add the remaining ½ squeezed lemon, and cook the chicken on all sides until golden brown for about 35 minutes. Add the red wine and continue to cook for several minutes before adding the water. Bring to a boil and reduce heat to low. Add the cinnamon stick, cloves, turmeric, onion, garlic cloves, and cardamom. Cover and cook on low heat for 1 hour and 45 minutes to 2 hours and 15 minutes. Keep covered and save the liquid chicken stock for the rice and ground meat mixture.

4. **Preparing the rice and ground meat mixture:** Rinse the rice, drain well, and set aside. Using a deep skillet, heat the remaining 1½ tablespoons of olive oil. Add the ground meat and cook on medium-high. Use a wooden spoon to break up the meat as it is cooking. Add the remaining 1 teaspoon of cinnamon powder, 1 teaspoon of allspice, 1 teaspoon of sea salt, and 1 teaspoon of black pepper. Cook the meat until it turns medium brown. Add ½ cup of the pine nuts and brown for a few minutes. Add the rice to the skillet. Stir for several minutes to combine. Pour 3 ½ cups of the prepared chicken stock into the skillet and stir. If there is insufficient chicken stock left, add water instead. Bring to a low boil and reduce heat. Cover and cook on low heat for 25 to 35 minutes.

5. **Preparing the toasted almond and pine nut topping:** In a small skillet on medium heat, add the sunflower oil and butter. Stir in the almonds. As the almonds begin to change color, add the remaining ½ cup of pine nuts. Continue to toss the almonds and pine nuts in the skillet until both are light golden.

May serve the chicken and rice separately or with the chicken over the rice and meat mixture. If serving together, pour the rice and meat mixture onto a large platter, placing the cooked chicken on top. Garnish with the prepared almond and pine nut topping. Serve warm.

Cook's secret: Cook the spiced chicken on all sides until golden brown.

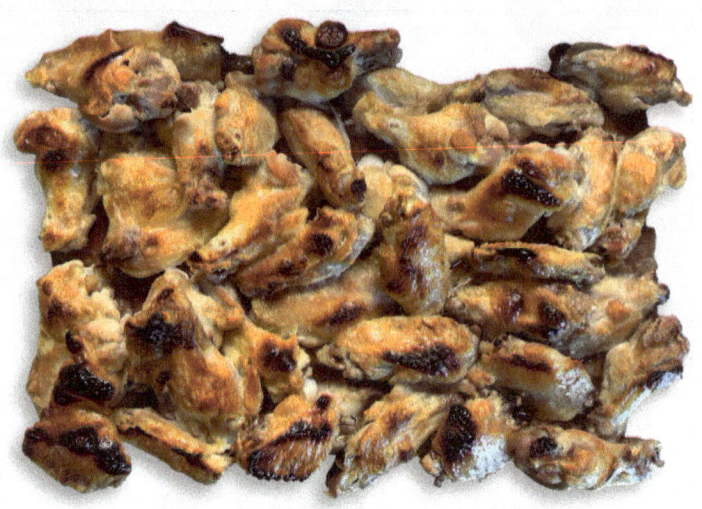

LEBANESE CHICKEN WINGS

Serves 2–4
Total time (preparation & cooking):
1 hour, 30 minutes

nutritional information per serving (6.6 oz.)

Cal 180 **Fat** 10g (sat 2.7g) **Chol** 40mg **Carbs** 9g **Sugars** 4g **Protein** 15g **Fiber** 2g **Sodium** 1198mg **Vit. A** (31% DV) **Vit. C** (47% DV) **Calcium** (8% DV) **Iron** (9% DV)

INGREDIENTS

- ½ pound cut chicken wings (split into drumstick and wing flat sections)
- ½ cup white distilled vinegar
- ¾ teaspoon baking powder
- 2 teaspoons table salt
- 3 medium tomatoes, finely chopped
- 1¼ teaspoons tomato paste
- 5 garlic cloves, peeled and mashed
- 1 tablespoon fresh ginger, finely chopped
- ½ fresh hot red pepper, finely chopped with seeds removed
- 1 cup fresh cilantro, finely chopped
- 1 teaspoon liquid yellow mustard (may substitute with 1 teaspoon of dried mustard)
- 1 tablespoon soy sauce
- 1 lemon, freshly squeezed
- 1 teaspoon paprika
- ¾ teaspoon dried oregano
- ½ teaspoon black pepper, coarsely ground
- ¼ teaspoon white pepper, finely ground
- ¼ teaspoon cayenne

INSTRUCTIONS

1. **Broiling the chicken wings:** Wash the chicken wings with the white distilled vinegar and 1 teaspoon of the table salt. Rinse with water and pat dry with a paper towel. Rub the dry wings with the baking powder and ½ teaspoon of table salt, coating evenly. Place the wings in a large rectangular baking dish about 2 inches deep. Broil in the oven on high for 10 to 12 minutes, or until they turn golden brown. Remove from the oven and discard any chicken juices or drippings from the baking dish. Flip the wings over and broil on the other side for 10 to 12 minutes. Remove from the oven, discard any juices, and set aside.

2. **Preparing the tomato sauce:** Place the remaining ½ teaspoon of table salt, tomatoes, tomato paste, garlic, ginger, hot red pepper, cilantro, mustard, soy sauce, lemon, paprika, oregano, black pepper, white pepper, and cayenne in a food processor or blender. Pulse to gently combine the ingredients. Transfer to a saucepan and cook on low heat for 12 to 15 minutes, stirring occasionally. Remove from the heat and set aside.

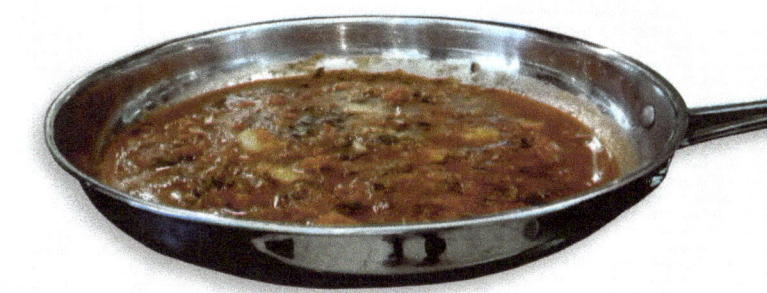

3. **Baking the chicken wings:** Use a paper towel to wipe off any chicken juices that may have collected in the baking dish. Pour the prepared tomato sauce over the wings, tossing to evenly coat. Return the wings to the oven and bake at 400°F for about 20 to 25 minutes. Remove from the oven and cover for 10 minutes before serving. Serve hot or warm.

Best served as is.

Cook's secret: Dry rub the wings with baking powder and salt before broiling, and discard the chicken juices.

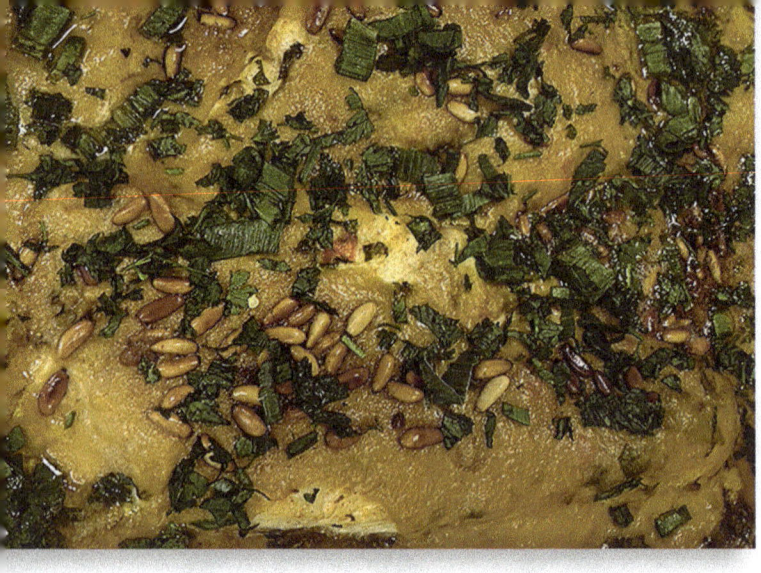

SPICY FISH
(SAMAKI HARRA)

Serves 4–6
Total time (preparation & cooking): 1 hour

nutritional information per serving (14 oz.)	**Cal** 785 **Fat** 58.7g (sat 8.6g) **Chol** 99mg **Carbs** 30g **Sugars** 5g **Protein** 42g **Fiber** 8g **Sodium** 1561mg **Vit. A** (9% DV) **Vit. C** (74% DV) **Calcium** (28% DV) **Iron** (35% DV)

INGREDIENTS

- 2 pounds wild-caught white fish (may substitute with frozen white fish, thawed)
- ½ cup extra-virgin olive oil
- ¾ cup lemon juice (freshly squeezed or bottled)
- ½ bunch fresh cilantro (about 1 cup)
- 1 tablespoon table salt
- 1 medium onion, chopped
- 6 large garlic cloves, peeled and mashed
- 1 cup tahini (sesame paste)
- ½ cup orange juice, freshly squeezed
- 1 fresh hot red pepper, diced
- ¼ teaspoon cayenne
- 2 tablespoons water
- 2 loaves pita bread (optional)

Nut topping

- 2 tablespoons sunflower oil
- 2 tablespoons unsalted butter
- ½ cup raw almonds, peeled and whole
- ½ cup pine nuts, whole

INSTRUCTIONS

1. **Preparing the fish:** Preheat the oven to 350ºF. Rinse the fish in cold water and set aside. Coat a large rectangular baking dish with ¼ cup of the olive oil. Place the fish in the baking dish and add ¼ cup of the lemon juice, fresh cilantro, and ½ tablespoon of the table salt. Bake the fish for 35 minutes. As the fish is baking, proceed to the next steps.

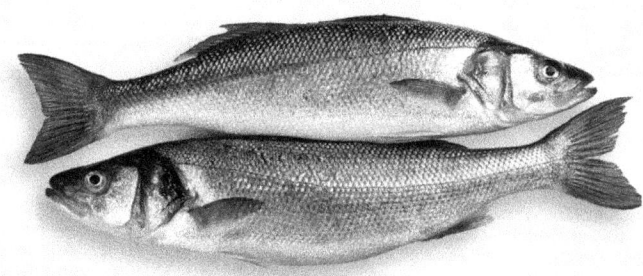

2. **Preparing the tahini sauce:** Place the remaining ¼ cup of olive oil in a small skillet. Add the onion and sauté for 4 to 5 minutes on medium heat. Stir in 3 of the garlic cloves and cook together for 3 minutes, or until the garlic turns a light golden brown. Set aside.

    In a saucepan on medium heat, add the tahini and orange juice. Stir well to combine. Add the hot red pepper and cayenne. Continue to stir while adding the remaining ½ cup of lemon juice, ½ tablespoon of table salt, and 3 garlic cloves. Add the water to create the desired thickness and consistency. Cook for 10 minutes. Stir in the prepared onion and garlic from the skillet. Cook together in the saucepan for another 5 minutes. Set aside.

3. **Preparing the nuts:** In a separate small-size skillet, heat up the sunflower oil and butter. Add the almonds and cook on low heat. After several minutes, or when the almonds begin to change color, stir in the pine nuts. Once the almonds and pine nuts are lightly browned, turn off the heat and set aside.

4. **Putting it all together:** Pour the prepared tahini sauce over the cooked fish, coating the fish evenly. Top with the roasted almonds and pine nuts. If serving with pita bread, toast the pita in a preheated oven at 375ºF for several minutes, or until it turns golden brown.

May also be served with fried pita bread.

Cook's secret: Use orange juice and lemon juice in the tahini sauce.

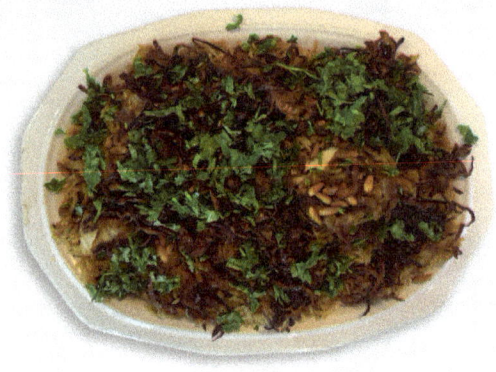

LEBANESE FISH WITH RICE
(SAYADIYA)

Serves 4–6

Total time (preparation & cooking): 1 hour, 50 minutes

---

nutritional information per serving (13.4 oz.) — **Cal** 666 **Fat** 46.9g (sat 7.9g) **Chol** 81mg **Carbs** 32g **Sugars** 5g **Protein** 40g **Fiber** 11g **Sodium** 619mg **Vit. A** (25% DV) **Vit. C** (30% DV) **Calcium** (10% DV) **Iron** (48% DV)

INGREDIENTS

Fish baste

- 3 garlic cloves, peeled and mashed
- ¼ teaspoon black pepper, coarsely ground
- ½ teaspoon paprika
- 2 tablespoons extra-virgin olive oil
- ½ teaspoon table salt

Fish

- 2 pounds wild-caught white fish, or about 4 white fish fillets with head (e.g., snapper, grouper, cod, or sea bass)
- 6 tablespoons vegetable oil (preferably sunflower oil)
- 5 medium onions, diced
- 4 garlic cloves, peeled and sliced
- 3 cups water
- 1 teaspoon fresh ginger, finely chopped
- 1 cinnamon stick
- 7 cardamom, whole
- 1 teaspoon cloves, ground
- 1½ cups white basmati rice, washed and drained
- 1½ teaspoons paprika
- 1 teaspoon coriander, ground
- 1 teaspoon black pepper, coarsely ground
- 1 teaspoon cumin, ground
- ½ teaspoon table salt
- ½ teaspoon saffron
- 3 tablespoons extra-virgin olive oil
- ½ cup Italian flat parsley, chopped and rinsed for garnish

Pine nut topping

- 1 tablespoon extra-virgin olive oil
- 1 tablespoon salted butter
- 4 tablespoons pine nuts, whole

INSTRUCTIONS

1. **Preparing the fish baste:** In a small bowl, combine the garlic, black pepper, paprika, olive oil, and table salt. Stir together and set aside the fish baste.

2. **Preparing the fish:** Rinse the fish in cold water and place on a large plate. Pat dry with a paper towel. Remove the skin, bones, and head. Discard the bones and set aside the fish head for the rice. Cut the fish into long fillet pieces and coat the fish on both sides with the fish baste. Cover the plate with plastic wrap and refrigerate until ready to fry.

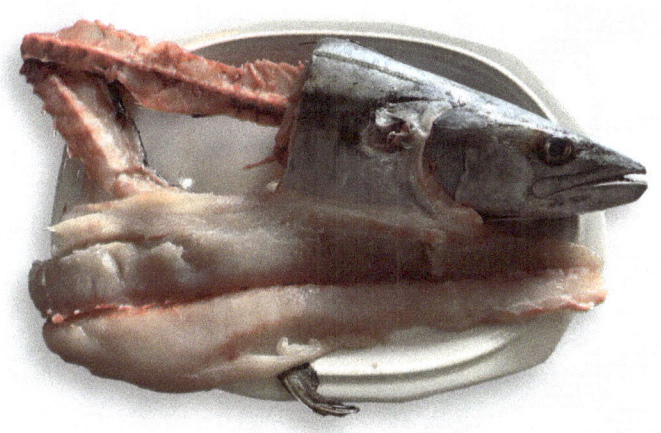

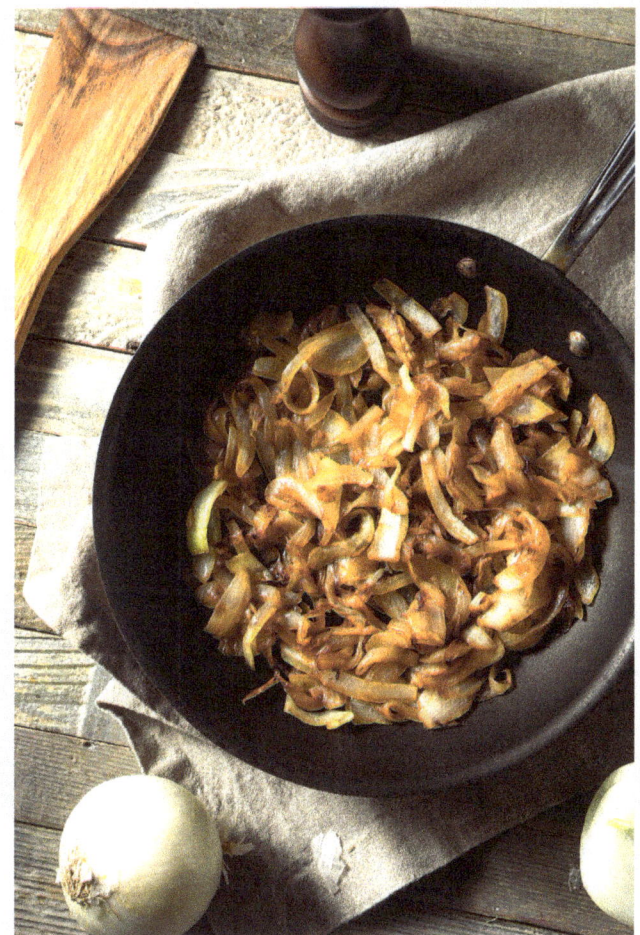

3. **Preparing the caramelized onions and garlic:** In a large skillet, heat the vegetable oil. Add the onions and sauté until well caramelized. Remove about 3 tablespoons of the caramelized onions for garnish and set aside. Stir in the garlic cloves and sauté with the onions for 3 minutes. Remove skillet from the heat and set aside.

MEAT, POULTRY & FISH | 83

4. **Preparing the fish stock for the rice:** In a large saucepan or stockpot, bring the water to a low boil. Add the ginger, cinnamon stick, cardamom, cloves, and fish head. Cook covered for 20 to 25 minutes on medium heat. Drain the stock from the saucepan, retaining 2½ cups of stock for cooking the rice. If there is insufficient stock left, use water instead. Discard the fish head and cinnamon stick.

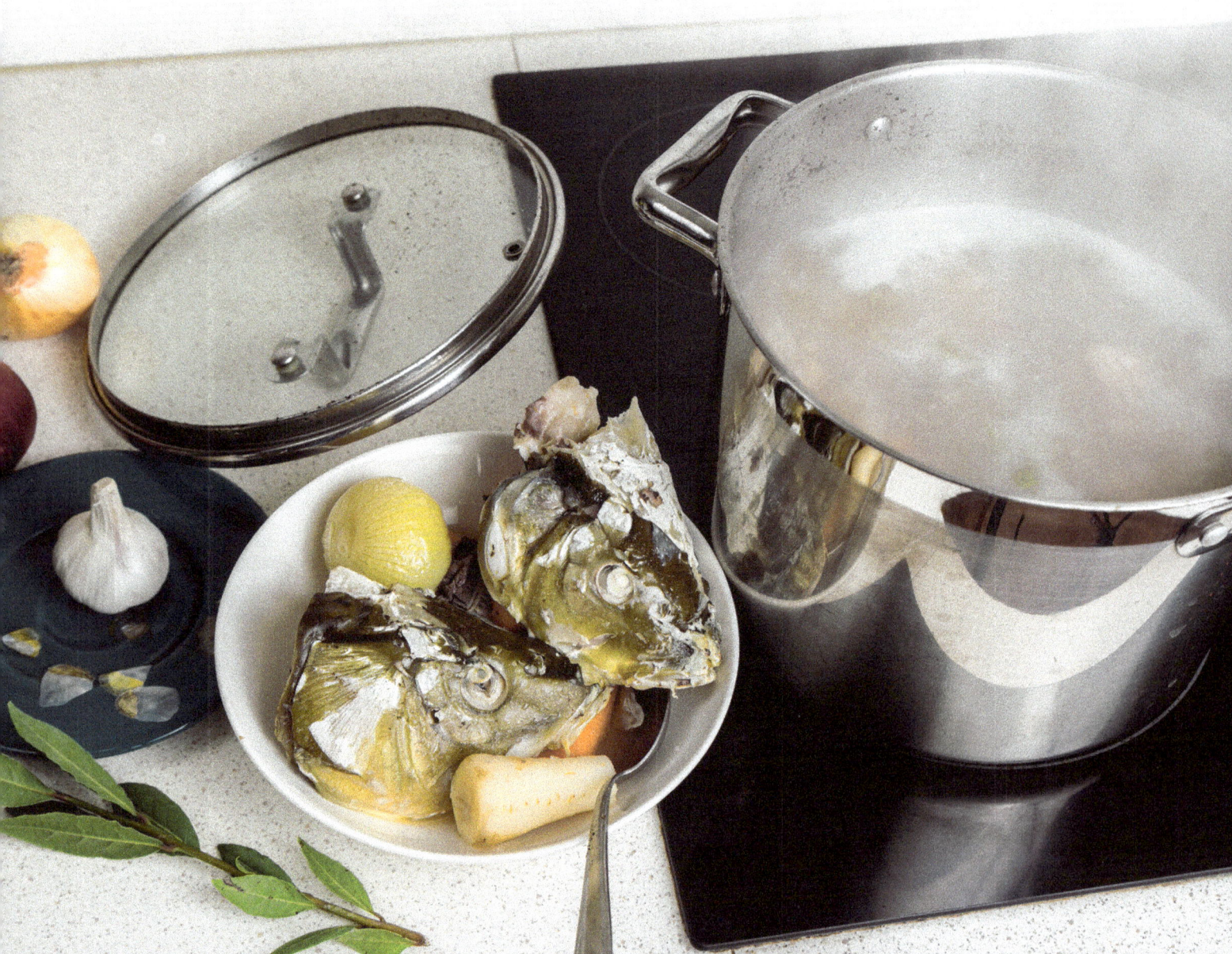

5. **Preparing the rice:** In a separate medium saucepan, bring the retained fish stock to a low boil on medium-high heat. Add the rice to the saucepan. Combine the paprika, coriander, black pepper, cumin, and table salt in a small bowl. Add the combined spices to the saucepan with rice. Immediately reduce heat to low. Stir in the saffron and the prepared caramelized onions and garlic. Cover and cook for 20 minutes, or until the rice is tender. Add more water if needed to cook the rice.

6. **Preparing the toasted pine nut topping:** In a separate, small-size skillet, heat the olive oil and butter. Stir in the pine nuts and sauté on low-medium heat for 5 minutes, or until the pine nuts turn light brown. Set aside.

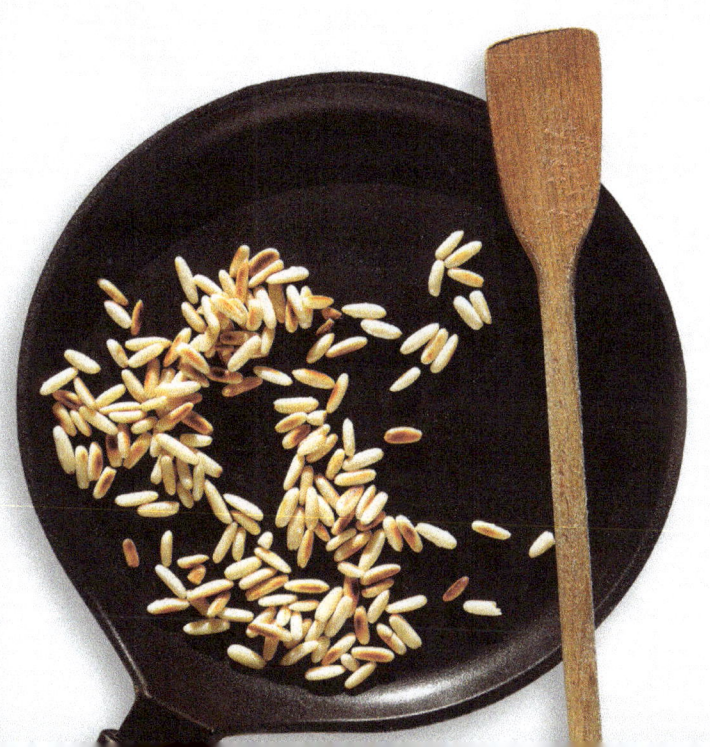

7. **Frying the fish fillets:** Remove the fish fillets from the fridge. In a medium frying pan or skillet, add the olive oil. Fry the fish fillets on medium heat for 5 to 6 minutes on each side, or until the fish is cooked. Remove from the heat.

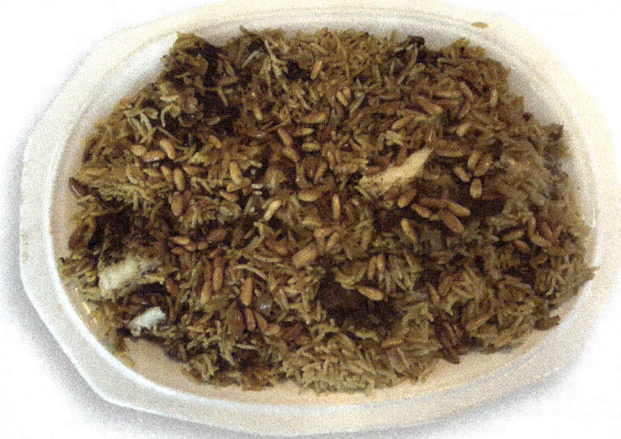

8. **Putting it all together:** Pour the prepared rice onto a large serving plate and arrange the fish fillets on top. Add the caramelized onions set aside for garnish. Finish with the prepared pine nut topping and sprinkle the parsley on top.

Best served as is.

Cook's secret: Use caramelized onions and saffron for flavor.

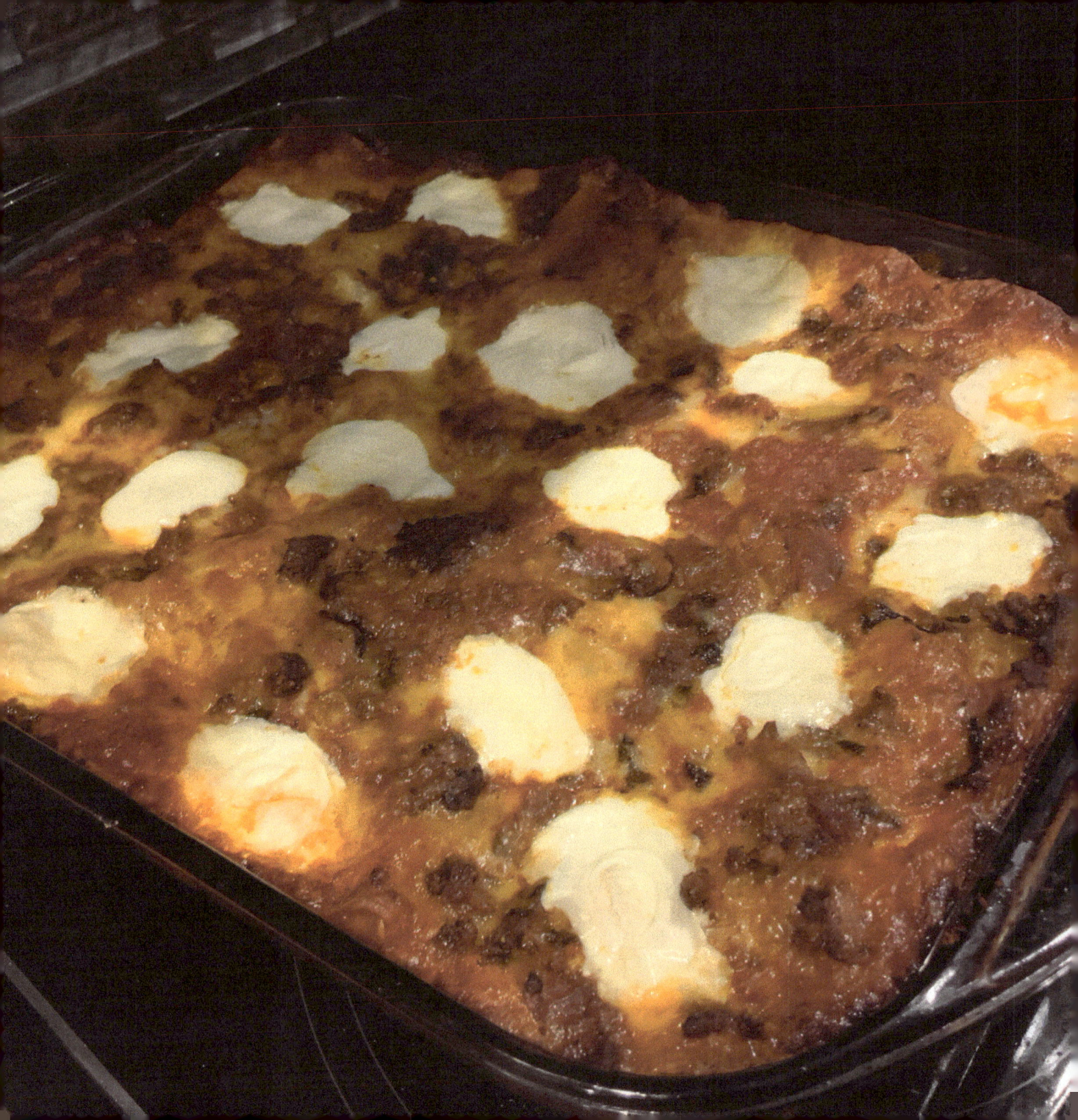

Fusion Dishes

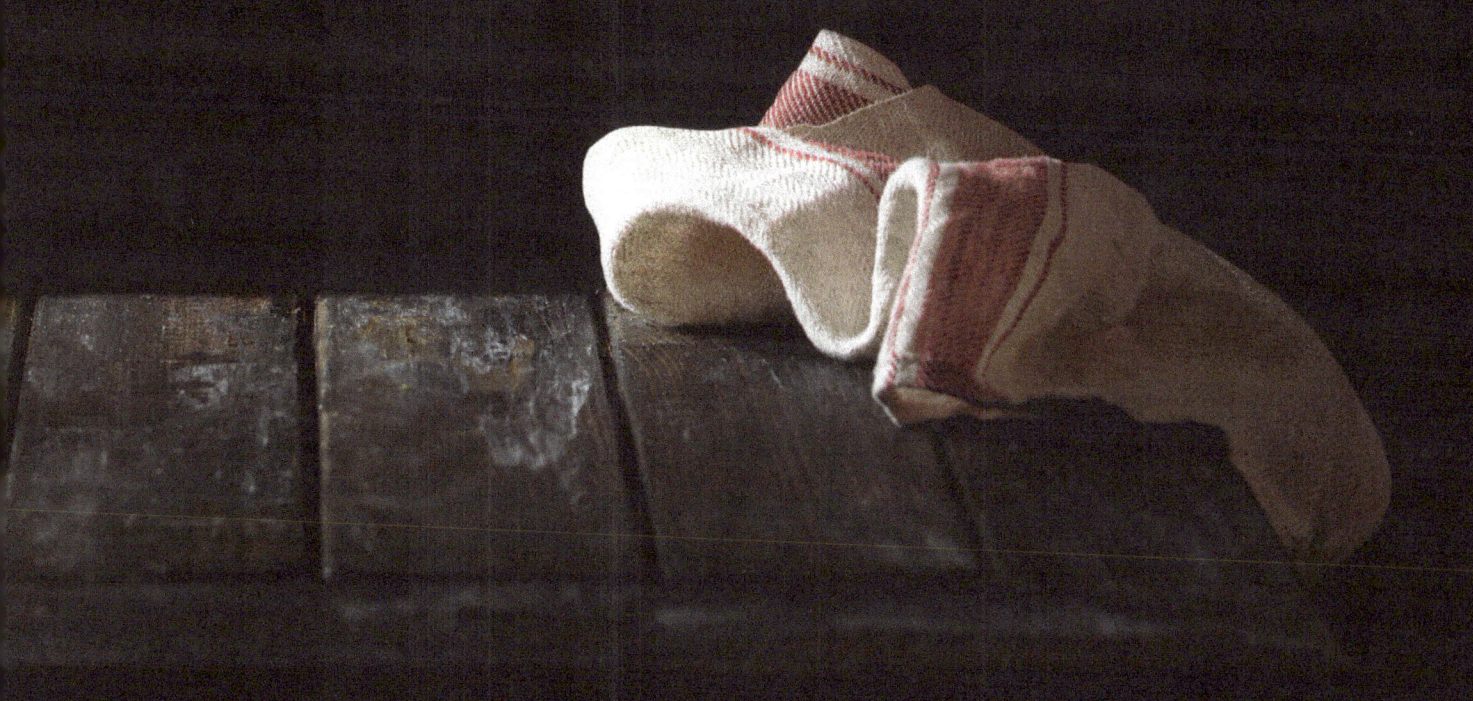

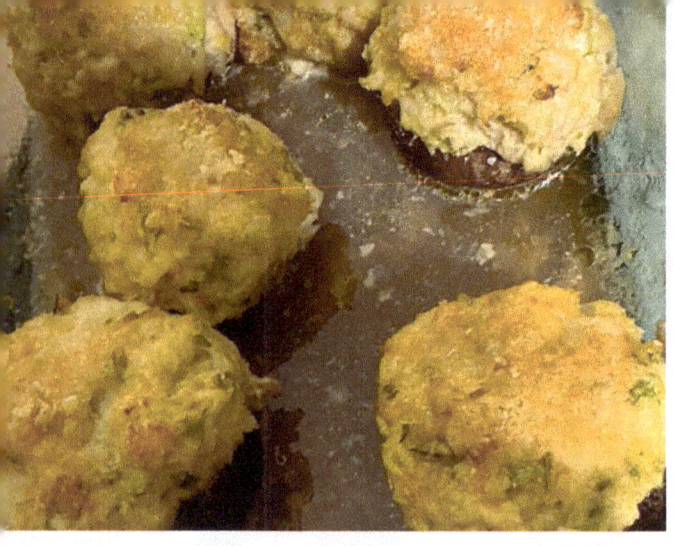

STUFFED MUSHROOMS

Serves 4
Total time (preparation & cooking):
1 hour, 40 minutes

---

nutritional information per serving (9.1 oz.)

Cal 279 **Fat** 15.6g (sat 7.3g) **Chol** 89mg **Carbs** 14g **Sugars** 4g **Protein** 22g **Fiber** 2g **Sodium** 1778mg **Vit. A** (16% DV) **Vit. C** (35% DV) **Calcium** (26% DV) **Iron** (9% DV)

INGREDIENTS

8	cups water
1	teaspoon table salt
1	bay leaf
1½	pounds fresh crab claws (may substitute with 10 ounces of canned crabmeat or canned shrimp)
15	large whole white mushrooms
1	teaspoon extra-virgin olive oil
2	tablespoons unsalted butter
3	scallions, very finely chopped
1	tablespoon white onion, very finely chopped
1	celery stick, finely chopped
3	tablespoons red bell pepper, very finely chopped
1	garlic clove, peeled and mashed (optional)
3	tablespoons bread crumbs
3	tablespoons mayonnaise
¼	teaspoon cayenne
1	lemon, freshly squeezed
¾	cup grated Parmesan cheese

INSTRUCTIONS

1. **Preparing the crab:** In a large stockpot or rondeau with about a five-quart capacity, bring the water to a boil. Add ½ teaspoon of the table salt, the bay leaf, and the fresh crab claws. Boil for 2 minutes or slightly longer for meatier varieties. Do not overboil as the crabmeat will become chewy. Drain and let the crab cool. Use a nutcracker or mallet to gently crack the claws. Remove the meat with a pick or a paring knife. Discard any stray crab shells and pieces of cartilage. The ratio of meat to shell will vary, but the edible portion of crabmeat needs to be about 10 ounces. Place the crabmeat in a medium bowl and set aside.

2. **Preparing the mushrooms:** Wash the mushrooms in cool water to remove dirt. Pop the stems out by gripping the mushroom stem side up and using your thumb to push against the stem. If the stem does not pop out in one piece, carefully remove any stem parts. Finely chop the stems and set aside. Place the mushroom caps in a baking dish coated with the olive oil. The baking dish should be large enough to fit all the mushrooms side by side. Preheat the oven to 350ºF and bake for 10 to 15 minutes to soften the mushrooms and prepare for stuffing. Remove mushrooms from the oven and set aside.

3. **Preparing the mushroom stuffing:** In a medium saucepan, melt 1 tablespoon of the butter. Brush each mushroom cap with the butter until all the butter is used. Melt the remaining 1 tablespoon of butter in the same saucepan over low-medium heat. Add the chopped mushroom stems, scallions, white onion, celery, red bell pepper, and garlic clove (if desired). Sauté for 40 minutes, or until the vegetables are tender.

   Pour the contents of the saucepan into the medium-size bowl containing the prepared crab. Add the bread crumbs, mayonnaise, cayenne, lemon, and the remaining ½ teaspoon of table salt. Mix to combine and break up the crabmeat. Add the Parmesan cheese, leaving some to sprinkle on top of the mushrooms before baking.

4. **Baking the stuffed mushrooms:** Using a spoon, fill each prepared mushroom cap in the baking dish with the prepared stuffing. When finished, sprinkle some of the Parmesan cheese over each mushroom, adding more grated cheese if needed. Bake at 350ºF for 25 minutes, or until the cheese-topped crab stuffing is golden brown. Serve hot or warm.

Best served as is.

Cook's secret: Prebake the mushrooms to soften, and sauté the vegetables with butter.

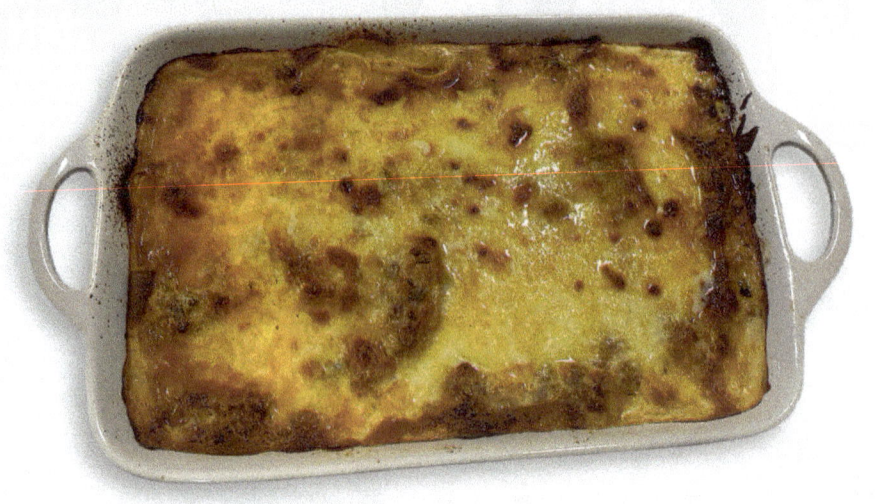

LEBANESE LASAGNA

Serves 5–6
Total time (preparation & cooking):
2 hours, 30 minutes

nutritional information per serving (25.8 oz.)
Cal 739 **Fat** 36.2g (sat 12.7g) **Chol** 154mg **Carbs** 48g **Sugars** 12g **Protein** 57g **Fiber** 5g **Sodium** 2242mg **Vit. A** (102% DV) **Vit. C** (148% DV) **Calcium** (67% DV) **Iron** (23% DV)

INGREDIENTS

- 4 tablespoons extra-virgin olive oil
- 1 onion, diced
- 3 garlic cloves, peeled and mashed
- 2 pounds ground lamb or beef (ground lamb preferred)
- ¼ teaspoon black pepper, coarsely ground
- ½ teaspoon cinnamon powder
- 1½ teaspoons dried oregano
- 1 teaspoon rosemary
- 1½ teaspoons sea salt
- 2 medium carrots, finely chopped
- 3 celery stalks, finely chopped
- ½ red bell pepper, finely chopped
- 1 fresh hot red pepper, finely chopped with seeds removed
- 2 cups fresh tomatoes, finely chopped
- 2 cups tomato juice, freshly squeezed
- 1 tablespoon tomato paste
- 1½ cups sliced portobello mushrooms
- 1 bunch fresh basil, finely chopped
- 1 tablespoon dried parsley
- 6 cups water
- 1 (9-ounce) package lasagna sheets, or 15 sheets
- 2 cups grated mozzarella cheese
- 1½ cups grated Parmesan cheese

INSTRUCTIONS

1. **Preparing the lasagna meat sauce:** In a large saucepot, heat the olive oil on low-medium. Add the onion and cook for 4 minutes. Add the garlic, cooking for another 2 to 3 minutes. Stir in the ground lamb and continue cooking on low-medium heat. After a few minutes, add the black pepper, cinnamon powder, oregano, rosemary, 1 teaspoon of the sea salt, carrot, celery, red bell pepper, and hot red pepper. Stir well to ensure that the ground meat is broken up and the vegetables and spices are thoroughly combined.

   Once the meat turns brown, stir in the chopped tomatoes, tomato juice, tomato paste, and sliced portobello mushrooms. Cook for 10 minutes, stirring occasionally. Stir in the fresh basil and dried parsley. Remove from the heat and set aside.

2. **Preparing the lasagna sheets:** In a large stockpot or rondeau with about a six-quart capacity, heat the water and add the remaining ½ teaspoon of sea salt. Bring to a boil and add the lasagna sheets. Cook for 5 minutes. Drain and set aside.

3. **Baking the lasagna meat sauce and pasta sheets:** In a large rectangular baking dish (13 by 9 inches), spread some of the lasagna meat sauce on the bottom, leaving enough meat sauce for three more layers. Place about 5 pasta sheets on the first layer and sprinkle ¾ cup of the grated mozzarella cheese on top. For the second layer, spread some of the lasagna meat sauce before adding 5 pasta sheets on top. Sprinkle ¾ cup of the grated mozzarella cheese and 1 cup of the grated Parmesan cheese on top of the second layer. For the third layer, add some of the lasagna meat sauce, spreading evenly, and place the remaining 5 pasta sheets on top. Sprinkle the remaining ½ cup of grated mozzarella cheese sauce on top of the third layer. For the fourth layer, add what is left of the lasagna meat sauce, spreading evenly. Do not place pasta sheets on the fourth and final layer. Sprinkle the remaining ½ cup of grated Parmesan cheese over the meat sauce. Bake in the oven on 350°F for 45 to 50 minutes.

   Best served as is.

   Cook's secret: Use generous portions of mozzarella and Parmesan cheese.

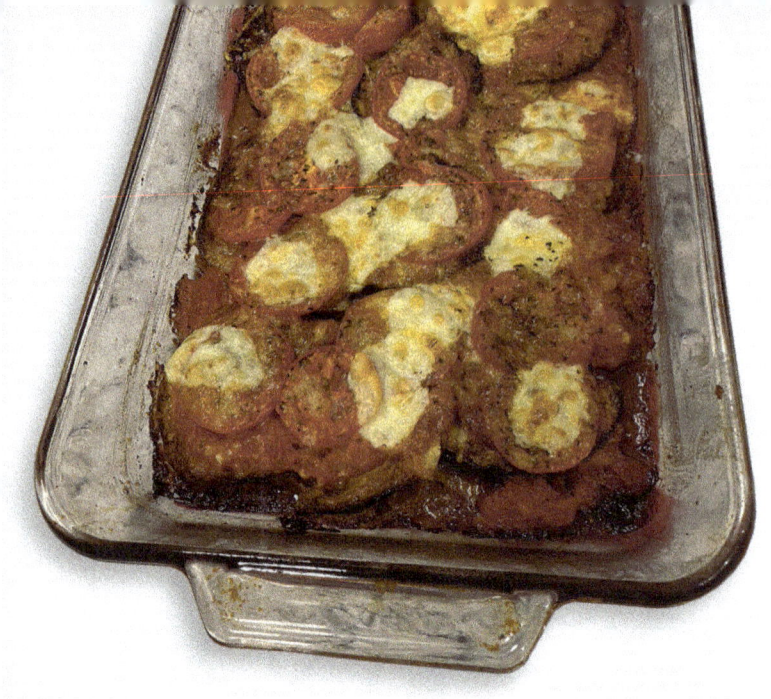

EGGPLANT PARMESAN

Serves 5–6
Total time (preparation & cooking):
1 hour, 50 minutes

---

nutritional information per serving (21.4 oz.) — **Cal** 488 **Fat** 9.3g (sat 4.1g) **Chol** 132mg **Carbs** 47g **Sugars** 15g **Protein** 46g **Fiber** 12g **Sodium** 1437mg **Vit. A** (51% DV) **Vit. C** (64% DV) **Calcium** (112% DV) **Iron** (21% DV)

INGREDIENTS

- 5 large tomatoes, diced
- 1 medium onion, chopped
- 3 garlic cloves, peeled and chopped
- ¼ teaspoon dried oregano
- ¾ cup fresh basil, finely chopped
- ¼ teaspoon cayenne (may substitute fresh hot red pepper)
- ¾ teaspoon black pepper, coarsely ground
- 1 teaspoon sea salt
- 2 large eggplants
- 3 eggs
- 1½ cups flour
- 1 pound fresh mozzarella cheese, sliced into thin disks
- 1 cup grated Parmesan cheese

INSTRUCTIONS

1. **Preparing the homemade tomato sauce:** In a food processor or blender, add the tomatoes, onion, garlic cloves, oregano, basil, cayenne, ½ teaspoon of the black pepper, and ½ teaspoon of the sea salt. Pulse together until the consistency is smooth like yoghurt. Place the ingredients in a saucepan and cook on low heat for 10 minutes, stirring occasionally. Set aside.

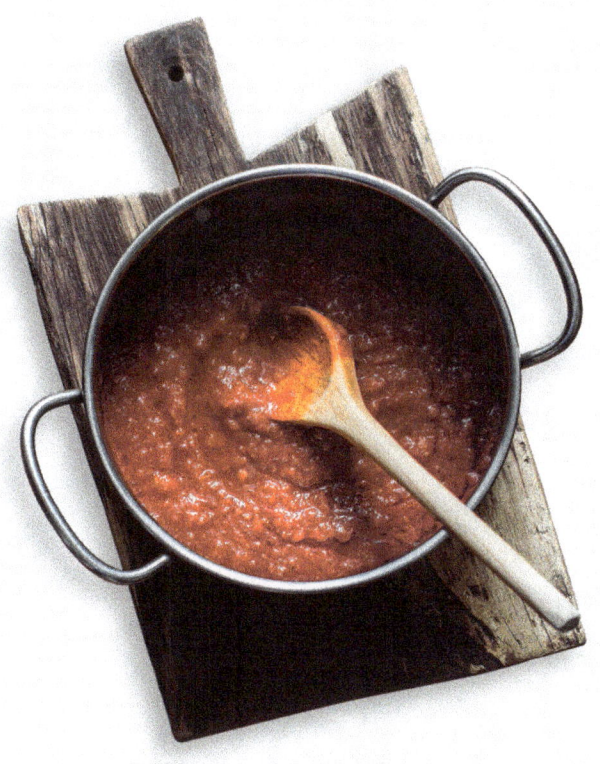

2. **Preparing the eggplant:** Preheat the oven to 350ºF. Slice the eggplant into disks about 1 inch thick. In a medium bowl, beat the eggs lightly and add the remaining ½ teaspoon of sea salt and ¼ teaspoon of black pepper. Fill a separate bowl with the flour. Dip each disk-shaped eggplant in the egg and then coat with flour. Place the eggplant on a greased baking pan. Bake for 10 to 15 minutes, or until light golden. Flip the eggplants over and cook for 10 to 15 minutes on the other side. Remove from the oven and set aside. Leave the oven on for the next step.

3. **Baking the eggplant and tomato sauce:** In a large rectangular baking dish about 2 inches deep, spread a small amount of the prepared tomato sauce on the bottom to prevent sticking. Place the prepared eggplant on the tomato-coated bottom, pouring the rest of the tomato sauce over the eggplant. Add the fresh mozzarella and Parmesan cheese on top. Bake at 350ºF for 25 to 30 minutes, or until the eggplant is cooked.

May be served as is or with rice.

Cook's secret: Use the homemade tomato sauce to bake the eggplant.

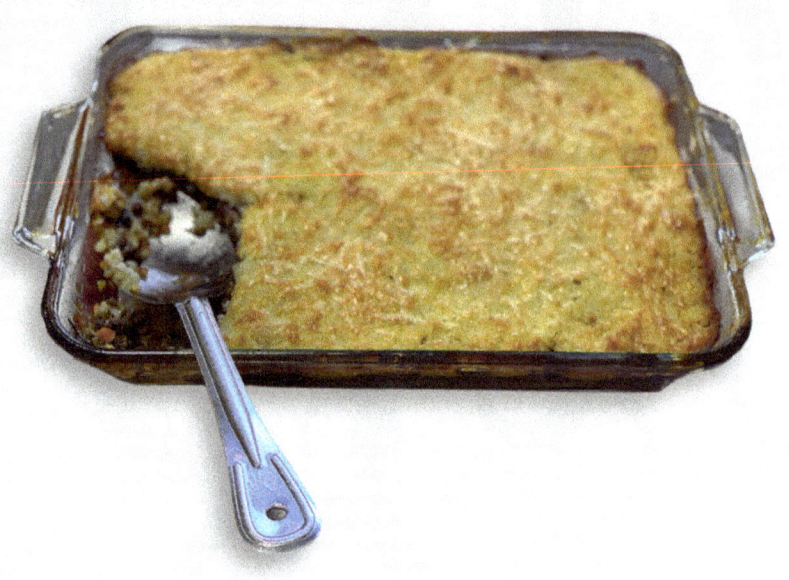

LEBANESE SHEPHERD'S PIE

Serves 6

Total time (preparation & cooking): 3 hours

---

nutritional information per serving (21.9 oz.) — **Cal** 871 **Fat** 38.3g (sat 13.4g) **Chol** 116mg **Carbs** 85g **Sugars** 8g **Protein** 47g **Fiber** 8g **Sodium** 1182mg **Vit. A** (93% DV) **Vit. C** (106% DV) **Calcium** (25% DV) **Iron** (40% DV)

INGREDIENTS

- 5 cups water
- 4 large russet potatoes, washed and unpeeled
- 3 tablespoons unsalted butter
- ¼ cup whole milk
- 1½ teaspoons table salt
- 3 cups water
- 1 cup medium-grain Egyptian white rice (may substitute with Arborio rice)
- 1 cup grated Parmesan cheese
- 5 tablespoons extra-virgin olive oil
- 1 large white onion, chopped
- 3 celery stalks, chopped
- 2 medium carrots, chopped
- 2 pounds ground lamb or beef (lamb preferred)
- 1 tablespoon soy sauce
- ½ teaspoon allspice, ground
- ½ teaspoon cinnamon powder
- ¼ teaspoon nutmeg, ground
- ½ teaspoon garlic powder
- ½ teaspoon cayenne
- 1 pound fresh peas (may substitute with frozen peas, thawed)
- ¼ cup red wine
- 1 tablespoon tomato paste

INSTRUCTIONS

1. **Preparing the potatoes:** In a large stockpot or rondeau with about a six-quart capacity, bring the water to a boil and add the potatoes. Boil for 30 to 35 minutes on low-medium heat, or until potatoes are cooked. Let the potatoes cool before peeling. Place the peeled potatoes in a large pan or bowl. Add 1 tablespoon of the butter, the milk, and ½ teaspoon of the table salt. Mash well to combine. Set aside.

2. **Preparing the rice:** In a medium saucepan, boil the water and ½ teaspoon of the table salt. Add the rice and the remaining 2 tablespoons of butter. Reduce heat to low. Simmer the rice for 15 to 20 minutes, or until it is partially cooked. Drain the rice and set aside.

3. **Combining the rice and potatoes to make the dough:** Add the cooked and drained rice to the mashed potatoes. Mix by hand, creating a dough-like blend. Add ½ cup of the grated Parmesan cheese and mix. Divide the dough into two equal portions. Set aside.

4. **Preparing the meat:** In a saucepan, heat 3 tablespoons of the olive oil on low. Add the onions, cooking for 3 to 4 minutes. Stir in the chopped celery and carrots. Add the ground meat, the soy sauce, allspice, cinnamon powder, nutmeg, garlic powder, cayenne, and the remaining ½ teaspoon of table salt. Mix to thoroughly combine spices and break up the ground meat. Add the peas and cook for 15 to 20 minutes. Stir in the red wine and tomato paste. Continue to cook for an additional 10 to 15 minutes. If needed, add ¼ cup of water to prevent the meat from drying out. Remove from the heat.

5. **Putting it all together:** Preheat the oven to 350°F. In a large baking dish, spread one portion of the rice and potato dough on the bottom. Make sure that the dough is all one thickness. Add the lamb filling, spreading it evenly over the dough. Spread the second portion of the dough evenly on a parchment sheet, or on the kitchen counter. Remove the dough from the sheet or counter and place on top of the lamb filling, spreading and shaping it to evenly cover the filling. Pour the remaining 2 tablespoons of olive oil on top of the dough. Sprinkle the remaining ½ cup of Parmesan cheese on top. Bake the shepherd's pie for 35 to 40 minutes. May broil for the last few minutes to brown the top.

Best served as is.

Cook's secret: Combine cooked rice and cooked potatoes to make the dough.

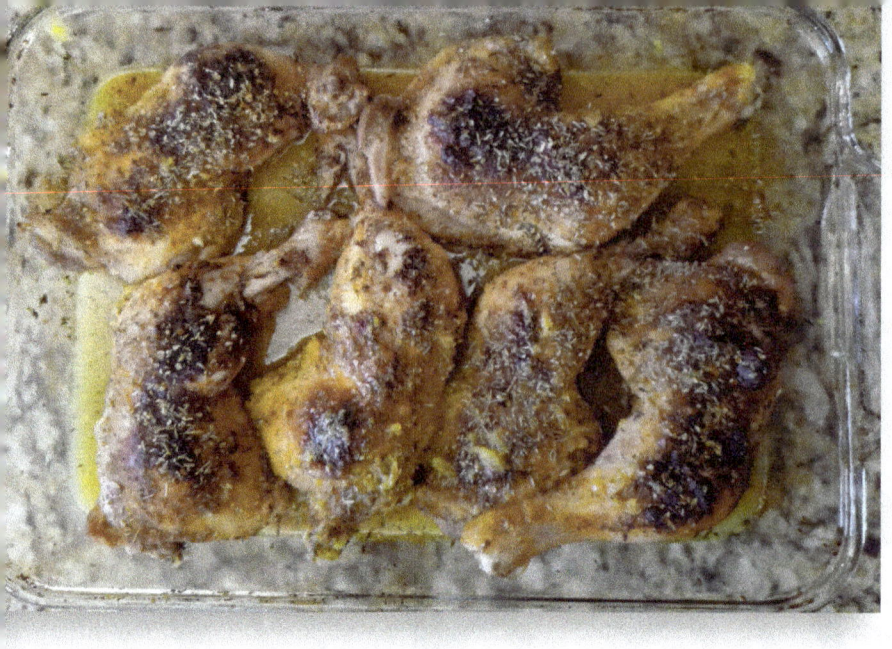

IKBAL'S CITRUS CHICKEN

Serves 4–6
Total time (preparation & cooking):
2 hours, 10 minutes

---

nutritional information per serving (9 oz.)

Cal 328 **Fat** 13.9g (sat 3.8g) **Chol** 192mg **Carbs** 13g **Sugars** 8g **Protein** 37g **Fiber** 2g **Sodium** 1313mg **Vit. A** (15% DV) **Vit. C** (75% DV) **Calcium** (6% DV) **Iron** (12% DV)

INGREDIENTS

- 2   Sumo Citrus oranges, squeezed (may substitute with blood oranges or tangerines)
- 2   navel oranges, squeezed
- 3   lemons, freshly squeezed
- 6   cups water
- 2   tablespoons table salt
- 2   pounds chicken legs, or about 6 pieces (bone-in and skin-on)
- 1½ teaspoons sea salt
- ½   teaspoon turmeric
- ¼   teaspoon cayenne
- 1½ teaspoons garlic powder
- 1½ teaspoons paprika
- 1½ teaspoons thyme
- 1   teaspoon dried oregano

INSTRUCTIONS

1. **Preparing the citrus sauce:** Add the squeezed Sumo Citrus oranges, navel oranges, and 2 of the squeezed lemons to a large bowl. Set aside.

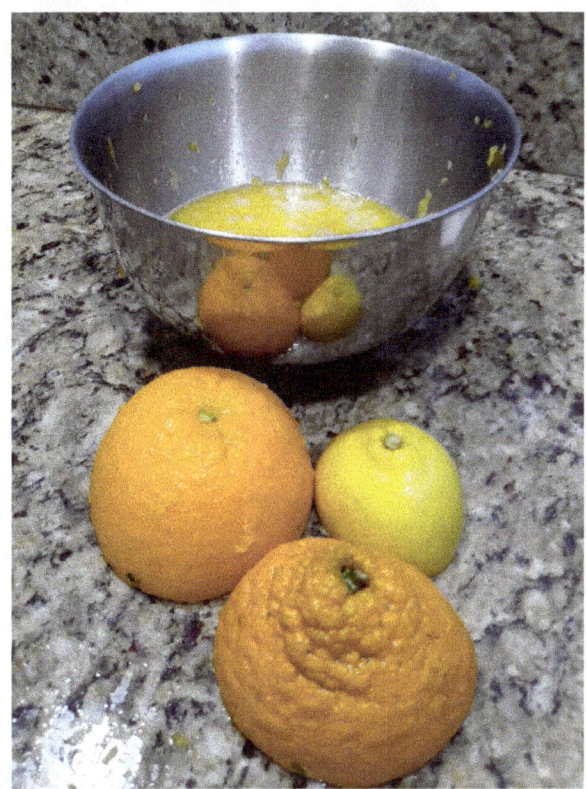

2. **Cleaning the chicken:** Fill a large food pan or bowl with the water. Add the table salt and the remaining squeezed lemon to the pan. Place the chicken legs in the pan and soak for 30 minutes. Drain the chicken with a colander and rinse off with cool water to remove salt. Cut off any excess skin from the chicken legs, leaving most of the skin on. Place the chicken legs in a large rectangular baking dish (13 by 9 inches) and set aside.

3. **Broiling the chicken:** Sprinkle the sea salt, turmeric, cayenne, 1 teaspoon of the garlic powder, 1 teaspoon of the paprika, and 1 teaspoon of the thyme over the chicken legs. Broil in the oven for 15 to 20 minutes on each side, or until it turns dark golden brown in color. Once the chicken legs are broiled evenly on both sides, remove from the oven. Allow to cool for 10 minutes. Discard the chicken juices from the pan. Pour the citrus sauce over the chicken legs. Spice the chicken legs once again, adding the oregano and the remaining ½ teaspoon of garlic powder, ½ teaspoon of paprika, and ½ teaspoon of thyme.

4. **Baking the chicken:** Bake the chicken legs (in the same baking dish) at 375ºF for 20 to 25 minutes, covering the baking dish with aluminum foil. Uncover and cook the chicken legs for another 20 minutes. Remove from the heat.

Best served as is.

Cook's secret: Use the citrus varieties to coat the broiled chicken before baking.

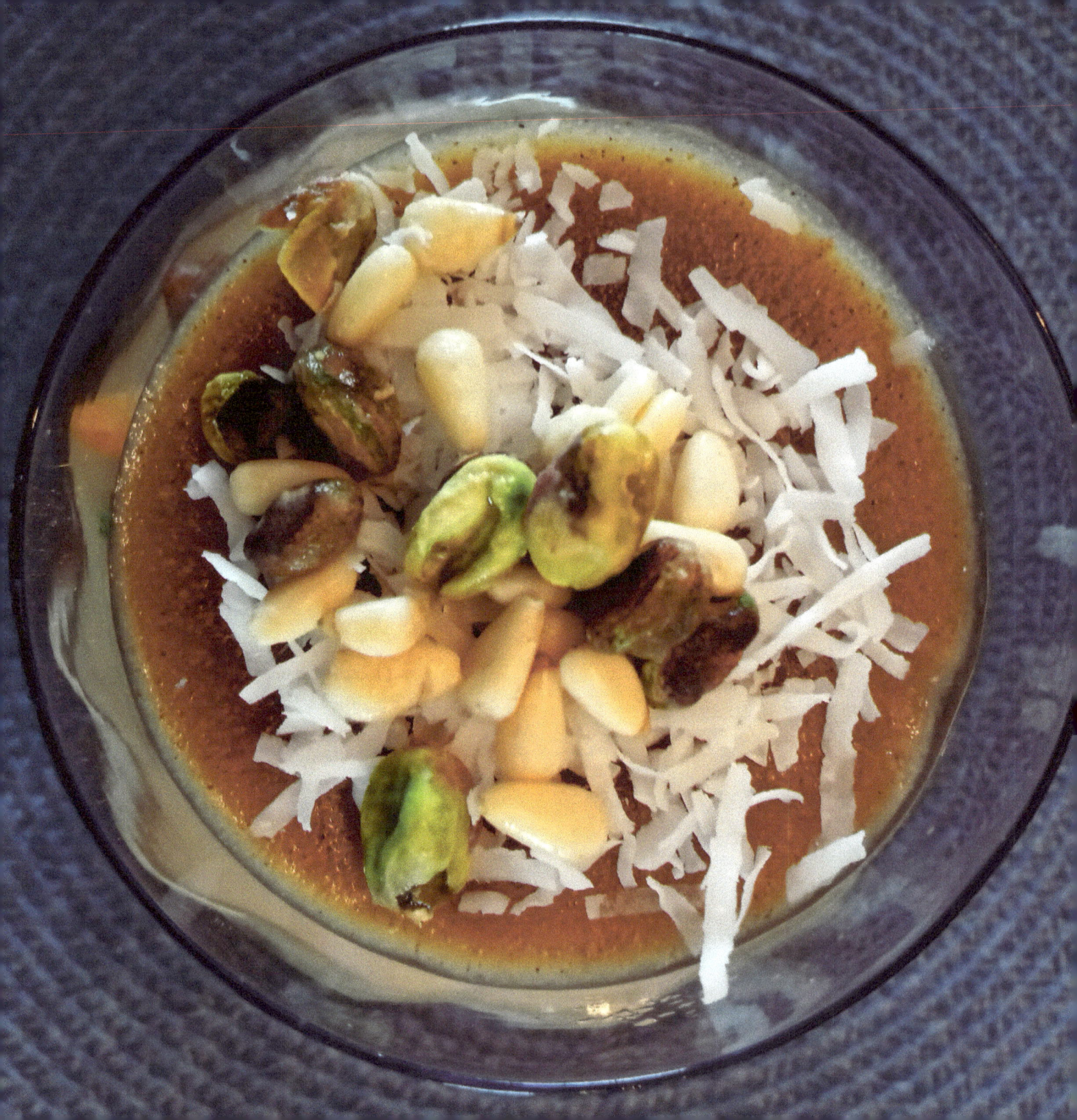

Desserts

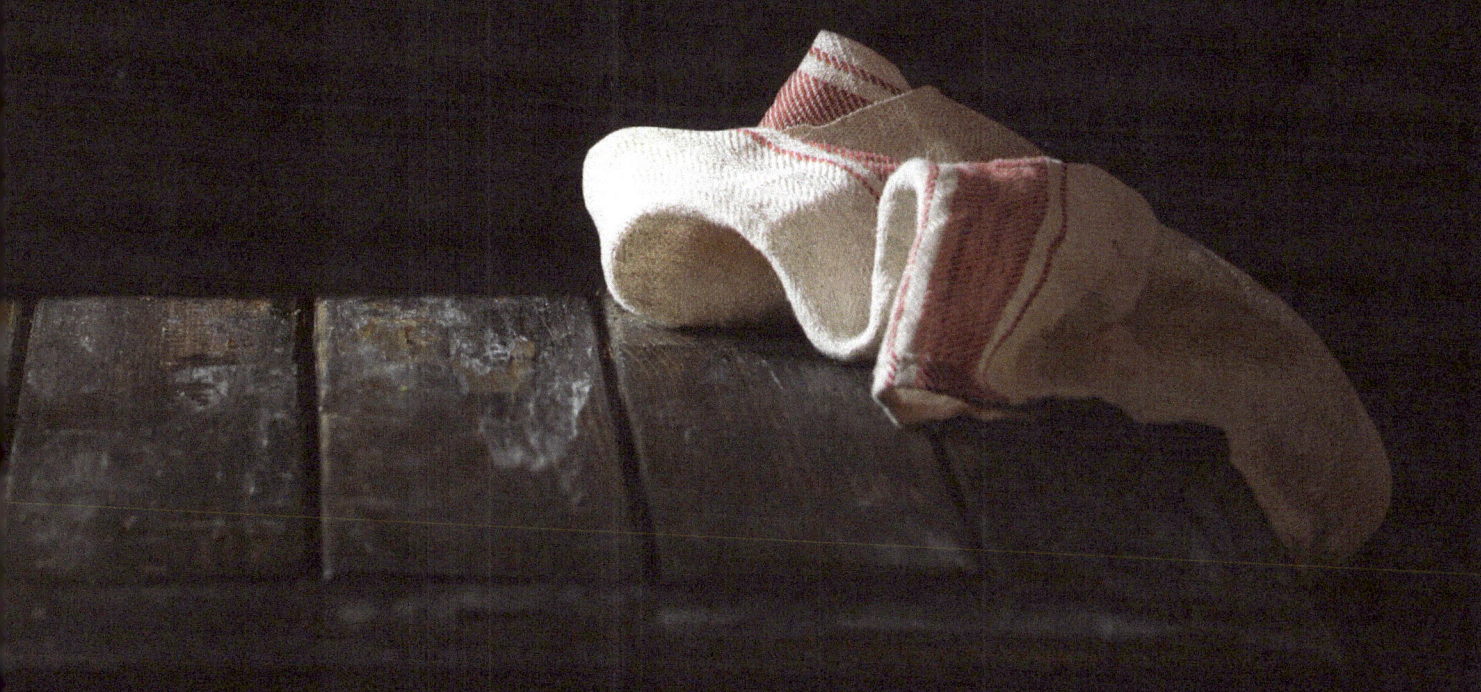

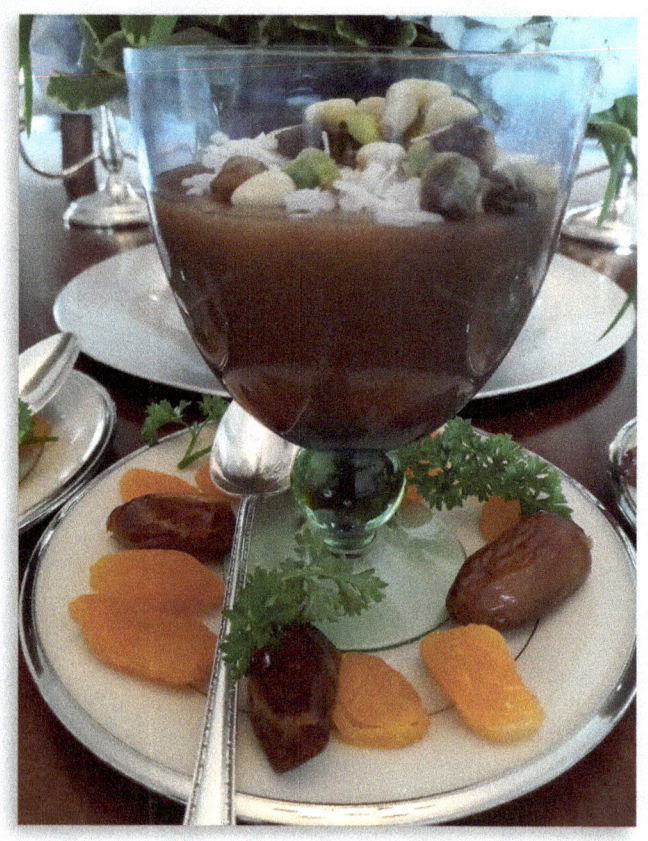

LEBANESE RICE PUDDING (MEGHLI)

Serves 6-8
Total time (preparation & cooking):
1 hour 25 minutes + 2 ½ hours soaking and refrigeration

nutritional information per serving (13.7 oz.)	**Cal** 500 **Fat** 22.7g (sat 9.3g) **Chol** 0mg **Carbs** 74g **Sugars** 52g **Protein** 6g **Fiber** 5g **Sodium** 12mg **Vit. A** (0% DV) **Vit. C** (2% DV) **Calcium** (8% DV) **Iron** (12% DV)

INGREDIENTS

8	tablespoons pine nuts, whole
8	tablespoons walnuts, whole
1	cup white rice flour
2	cups granulated sugar
1½	tablespoons cinnamon powder
½	teaspoon ginger powder
½	teaspoon dried greater galangal (*kholanjan*), ground (may substitute with 0.035 ounces dried greater galangal, whole)
½	teaspoon nutmeg, ground
1½	tablespoons anise, ground
2	tablespoons caraway, ground
9½	cups water
4	teaspoons pistachios, ground
8	tablespoons coconut, desiccated or shredded

INSTRUCTIONS

1. **Soaking the nuts:** Place the pine nuts and walnuts in separate bowls. Fill the bowls with enough cold water to cover the nuts. Soak for about 2 hours. Drain and set aside.

2. **Boiling the pudding:** In a large bowl, combine the rice flour, sugar, cinnamon powder, ginger powder, greater galangal, nutmeg, anise, and caraway. Gradually add the water and stir to combine. Pour the contents into a large saucepan or stockpot with about a six-quart capacity. Bring to a boil on medium heat, stirring constantly in the same direction using a wooden spoon or hand whisk. Continue to stir for the entire duration of cooking time.

   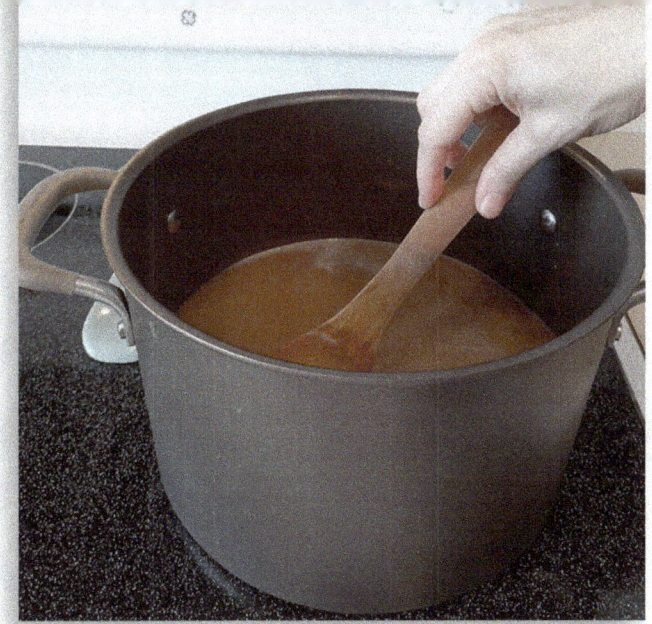

   After about 30 or 35 minutes, test to see if the pudding is done by holding up a spoonful of pudding over the stockpot, allowing it to drip off the spoon. If the pudding drips slowly off the spoon in long strands, it is done. If it is watery or runny and drips quickly, then continue to stir on medium heat until it thickens.

   When complete, immediately pour the hot pudding into about 8 small individual bowls. If using glass serving bowls, warm up the glass beforehand by rinsing it with 50% tap water and 50% boiling water to prevent cracking. Allow the pudding to sit for about 40 minutes before placing in the fridge to chill and thicken. Chill for at least 2 ½ hours.

3. **Garnishing the pudding:** Remove from the fridge and sprinkle ½ teaspoon of the pistachios over each bowl of pudding. To finish, top each bowl with 1 tablespoon of the coconut, 1 tablespoon of the soaked walnuts, and 1 tablespoon of the soaked pine nuts.

   Best served as is.

   Cook's secret: Stir the pudding constantly on medium heat and use pungent spices of dried cinnamon, ginger, greater galangal, anise, and caraway.

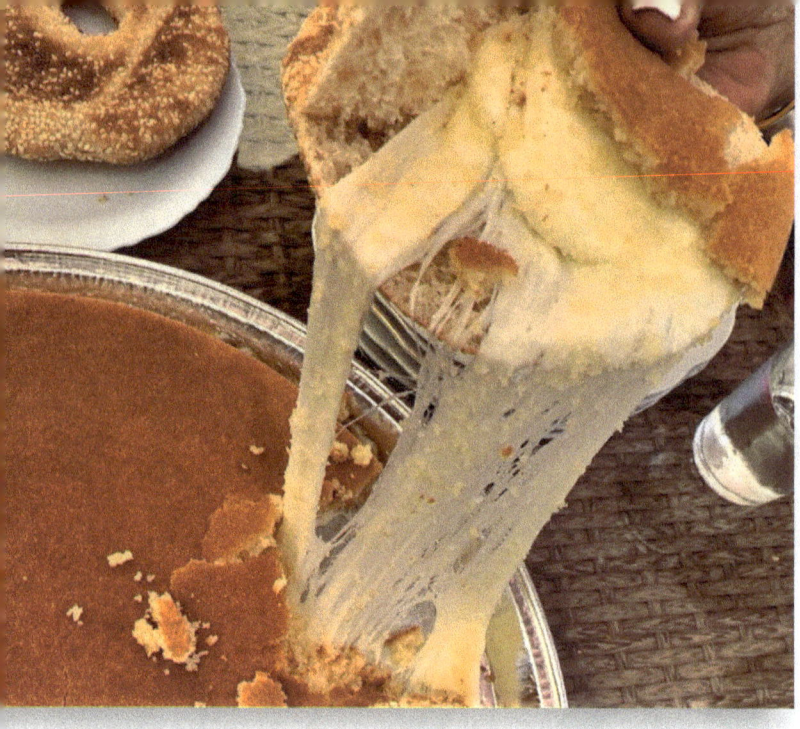

LEBANESE SWEET CHEESE PASTRY

(KNAFEH BI JIBN)

Serves 8-10
Total time (preparation & cooking):
1 hour 50 minutes

> nutritional information per serving (13.6 oz.) : **Cal** 738 **Fat** 18.6g (sat 11.2g) **Chol** 60mg **Carbs** 13g **Sugars** 8g **Protein** 37g **Fiber** 5g **Sodium** 812mg **Vit. A** (22% DV) **Vit. C** (0% DV) **Calcium** (114% DV) **Iron** (15% DV)

INGREDIENTS

- 2 cups semolina flour, coarsely ground
- 1¾ cups semolina flour, finely ground
- 2 sticks unsalted butter (8 ounces, or ½ pound), melted (may substitute with ghee or *samneh*)
- 6 tablespoons rose water
- 7 tablespoons orange blossom water
- 3 cups water
- 1¾ cups granulated sugar
- 1 teaspoon lemon juice (freshly squeezed or bottled)
- 2 pounds fresh mozzarella cheese
- 1 pound ricotta cheese

INSTRUCTIONS

1. **Preparing the pastry dough:** On a large flat tray, combine the coarsely ground semolina flour and 1 ½ cups of the finely ground semolina flour. Pour the butter over the semolina flour, saving about 3 teaspoons or ½ ounce for greasing the pan that will be used to bake the dough (unless using a nonstick pan or lining the pan with parchment paper). Add 2 tablespoons of the rose water and 3 tablespoons of the orange blossom water. Knead well by hand to combine the ingredients into a smooth, even dough. Cover with a towel and allow to sit for 30 minutes.

2. **Preparing the *attar* or sugar-based syrup:** In a large saucepan, combine the water, sugar, and lemon juice. Cook uncovered on low heat, stirring infrequently. Once the sugar dissolves, raise the heat to medium and stop stirring to prevent crystallization. Cook for 10 more minutes, or until the attar develops a thicker consistency. Remove from the heat and fold in 1 tablespoon of the rose water and 1 tablespoon of the orange blossom water. Set aside to cool.

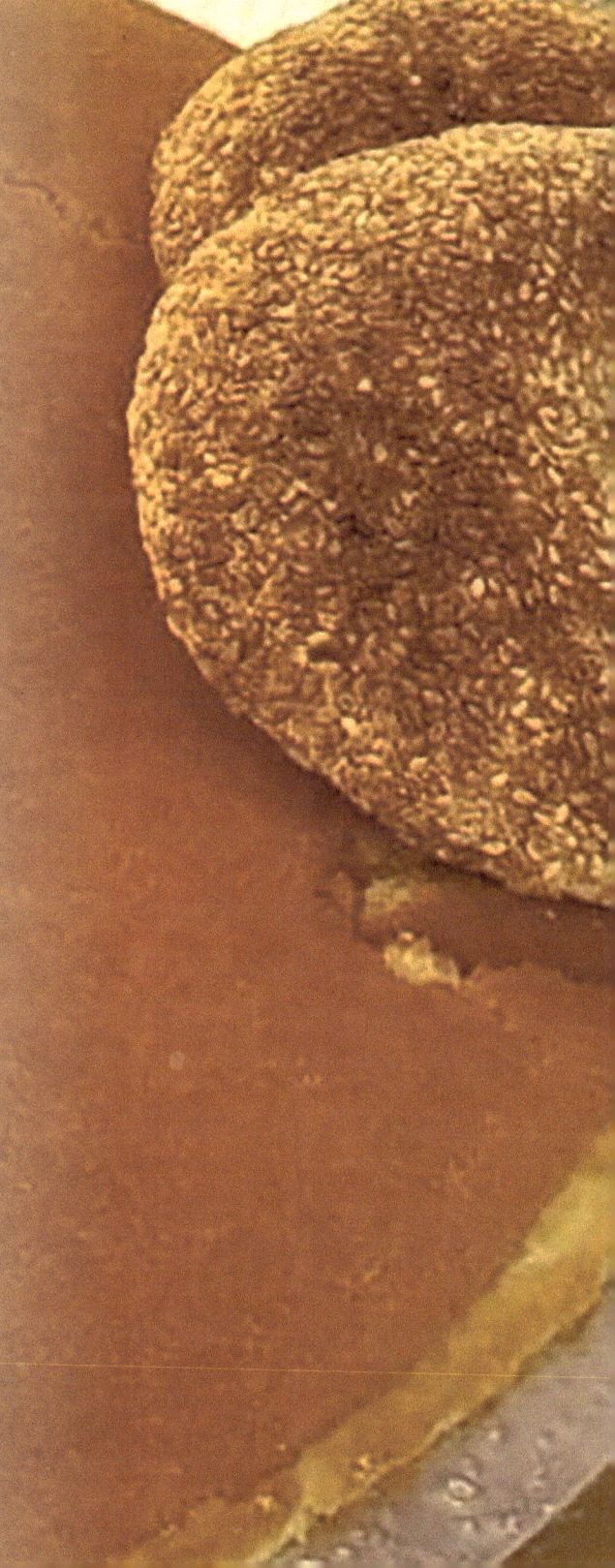

3. **Baking the pastry dough crust:** Grease a shallow, round baking pan with a thin layer of the saved butter to prevent sticking. The baking pan should be 12 or 14 inches in diameter and about 2 inches deep. Spread the prepared dough out evenly into a circle to fit the baking pan. Bake in a preheated oven at 350°F for 20 minutes, or until the dough crust is golden brown. Cover with aluminum foil to keep warm and set aside.

4. **Cooking the cheese:** In a separate large saucepan with the heat turned off, combine the mozzarella cheese and ricotta cheese. Add the remaining ¼ cup of finely ground semolina flour, 3 tablespoons of rose water and 3 tablespoons of orange blossom water. Stir with a wooden spoon to combine. Pour in ¼ cup of the prepared attar. Turn on the stove and cook on medium heat, stirring constantly. Cook for 10 to 15 minutes, or until the cheese is completely melted.

5. **Putting it all together:** Uncover the baked pastry dough and pour the melted cheese evenly over the dough, avoiding the outer edge of the crust. Place a shallow serving plate or tray that is a little larger than the round baking pan facedown over the pan. Using oven mitts or pot holders, grip the plate firmly over the pan. Once grip is secure, invert or flip the pan upside down in one swift motion so that the plate ends up on the bottom and the pastry dough ends up on top. Gently lower the plate onto a counter surface and then lift up to remove the pan. Drizzle the desired amount of attar over the dough. Serve warm.

May be served as is or stuffed inside sesame *kaak* bread (a popular Lebanese street bread).

Cook's secret: Use both coarsely ground and finely ground semolina flour to make the dough crust and cook the melted cheese with some of the attar.

www.ingramcontent.com/pod-product-compliance
Lightning Source LLC
Chambersburg PA
CBHW061406010526
44119CB00011B/271